Occupational Therapy for Older People

Christian Pozzi • Alessandro Lanzoni
Maud J. L. Graff • Alessandro Morandi
Editors

Occupational Therapy for Older People

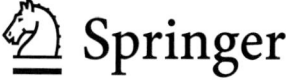 Springer

Editors
Christian Pozzi
University of Applied Sciences and Arts
SUPSI University of Applied Sciences
and Arts
Manno, Switzerland

Maud J. L. Graff
Radboud University Nijmegen
Nijmegen, The Netherlands

Alessandro Lanzoni
NODAIA Dementia Unit
Private Hospital Villa Igea
Modena, Italy

Alessandro Morandi
Department of Rehabilitation
and Aged Care
Hospital Ancelle
Cremona, Italy

Institute of Research and Parc
Sanitari Pere Virgili
Barcelona, Spain

ISBN 978-3-030-35730-6   ISBN 978-3-030-35731-3   (eBook)
https://doi.org/10.1007/978-3-030-35731-3

This Springer imprint is published by the registered company Springer Nature Switzerland AG
The registered company address is: Gewerbestrasse 11, 6330 Cham, Switzerland

Contents

Introduction

Marco Trabucchi and Stephanie Saenger

1.1 Geriatric Care Needs Different Professional Approaches: The Role of Occupational Therapists

Marco Trabucchi

I am honored to collaborate with this very important book, thus contributing to the diffusion of the profession of occupational therapist and to the increase of the general esteem for its role in the medical field. As president of Italian Psychogeriatric Association, I had many occasions to discuss with occupational therapists about the theoretical basis of the profession and its operative contents in the real world. Always I had the impression that our projects and the clinical programs were following a parallel route. Although starting from different basis, our reasoning was grounded on the deep persuasion of the centrality of patients and the consequent need to personalize any clinical approach. In particular, I was impressed in many occasions by the enthusiasm of occupational therapists, presenting their positions without any superficial declaration, but with the pride of having ideas deeply elaborated with the aim of producing peculiar results for the wellbeing of the old patient.

In the following points, I would like to briefly summarize some ideas (my personal and of the Italian Psychogeriatric Association) concerning the basis for an active role of occupational therapists in the care of the elderly:

M. Trabucchi
Italian Psychogeriatric Association, Brescia, Italy
e-mail: trabucchi.m@grg-bs.it

S. Saenger (✉)
COTEC (Council of Occupational Therapist for the European Countries), Karlsbad, Germany
e-mail: s.saenger@xs4all.nl

© Springer Nature Switzerland AG 2020
C. Pozzi et al. (eds.), *Occupational Therapy for Older People*,
https://doi.org/10.1007/978-3-030-35731-3_1

- Multidimensional Geriatric Assessment is the first act to perform when approaching an old person needing medical care. Occupational therapists usually incorporate this procedure in their everyday procedures.
- The recognition of multimorbidity and of different psychosocial factors interacting with health is the basis for the cure of the elderly, and for any successful intervention. This cultural attitude drives everyday practice of occupational therapists.
- Based on the recognition of the multiple origins of the loss of autonomy, which take place in the old age, any possible intervention needs to be founded on the collaboration of different professionals, each with his own heritage of knowledge and experience.
- In the different phases of a disease treatment and of rehabilitative actions each profession exerts its peculiar function, also assuming a leading role when needed. Thus also occupational therapists play a leading role when the main problem is the return to normal activities and the other professionals have only a collaborative function.
- Occupational therapists play a pivotal role when the goal is the return to daily living occupations at home. Moreover, their interventions are important also in nursing homes, where maintaining good level of autonomy is necessary to allow the participation of the various activities. Occupational therapies play a role also in institutions giving palliative care, when patients need to be able to defeat at the same time pain and inactivity.
- Occupational therapists before any intervention must understand the peculiar sense of life of the single patient, in absence of which all efforts to return to previous conditions are in vain. Understanding the scope of the existence of each person is of great help in performing single acts of cure, whose final target is to allow the realization of predefined objectives.
- The scopes of occupational therapy interventions are peculiar, since they range from a direct rehabilitative activity to the adaptation of life environments, to the education of caregivers and, in general, of the family and the community (this last point is of primary relevance, because society has an important collaborative function in facilitating the return of a single patient to the original role).
- In the modern society, characterized by an huge increase of the needs of the elderly, mostly due to the survival of persons who underwent an acute disease followed by a chronic one, it is increasing the role of professionals able to reduce the social burden induced by a large amount of citizens unable to behave independently in the activities to be performed in their own house and in the working and social activities.
- I am rather certain that in the future occupational therapy will increase its important role in the contemporary medical and social scenario; in fact we will need professionals able to direct the interventions on the elderly to a better insertion in the daily activities, avoiding the exclusion due a reduced physical or psychological function.

1.2   The Importance of Networks for Visibility and Availability of Occupational Therapy Across Europe

Stephanie Saenger

I am very pleased to be asked to write a part of the introduction of this important book. The editors have done a great work in bringing together authors and editors who have good reputations and networks across Europe and worldwide. It is also important that their network goes beyond the profession of occupational therapy.

The fact that I, as president of the Council of Occupational Therapist for the European Countries (COTEC), have been asked to write a part of this introduction is an acknowledgement of the power of networks and the work of COTEC in recent years. COTEC is the organization bringing European Occupational Therapy professional associations together, and I realize every day how international networks can strengthen the body of knowledge, the enthusiasm of professionals, the research and, in the end, the profession. Networks are very important in the process of professionalizing the individual, the profession, and organizations such as professional associations. Networks can create a "momentum" and this book is a good example of a momentum created by the energy, knowledge, and will to share and cooperate.

The power and importance of a network exceeds the sum of all the individuals.

Networks and NGO's like European Forum for Primary Care, ParkinsonNet, Community Occupational Therapy in Dementia (COTiD) EDOMAH (Dutch)/ COTID (European) networks, European Interdisciplinary Network on Psychosocial Interventions in Dementia (InterDem), European Delirium Association, International Association of Hospice and Palliative Care, European Public Health Association, World Family Doctors (WONCA), International Association of Hospice and Palliative Care (IAHPC), European Federation of the Associations of Dietitians (EFAD), Comité Permanent de Liaison des Orthophonistes/Logopedes de l'Union Européenne (CPLOL), European Region of the World Confederation of Physical Therapy (ER-WCPT), International Federation of Social Workers (IFSW), Horatio (Association of nurses in Mental Health). European Psychiatric Association (EPA), European Federation of Psychologists' Associations (EFPA), European Health Professionals Dialogue, WEMOS, are crucial to the process of implementing WHO-Europe resolutions.

Being a part of a European network empowers the professional and the profession. By talking to, and working with, professionals from another country, it is possible not only to learn new topics and skills, but also to see everybody's work and profession from another perspective. In occupational therapy the context is very important. With international networks one can identify the influence of the context on life, health, and social care. Europe, although one continent, has a lot of cultural, legal, financial, and political differences, which influence the perspective on health and healthcare, support to caregivers, and on the role and status of occupational therapy.

Occupational therapy has been growing in the last years (Fig. 1.1) and even the numbers of students in OT have increased showing the interest and the importance of this profession [1, 2].

However, there is still a variability across Europe and even terminology is important to exactly name the occupational therapy in different countries. Indeed in Europe a lot of different names in Europe (Table 1.1) are used for an occupational

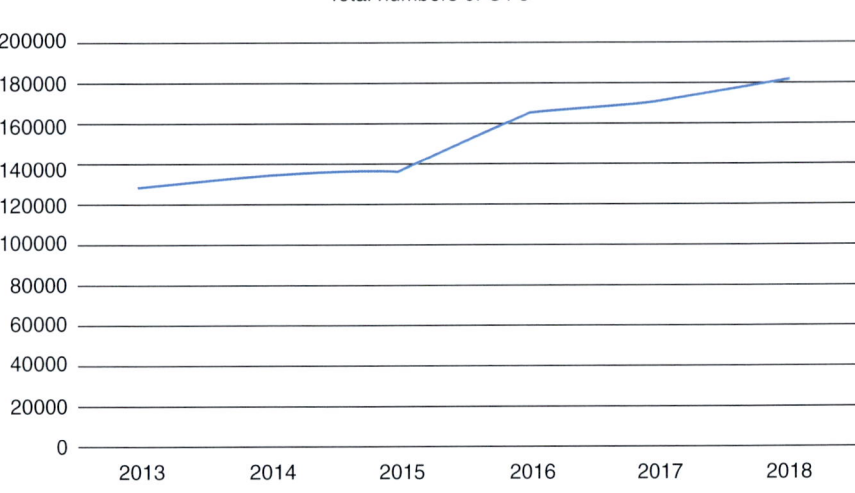

Fig. 1.1 The total number of occupational therapists in Europe from 2013 to 2018

Table 1.1 Terms used to name occupational therapy across Europe	
	Ergotherapeut
	Radni terapeut
	Diplomirani delovni terapevt
	Iðjuþjálfi
	Ergoterapeut
	Toimintaterapeutti
	Ergothérapeute
	Terapeuta ocupacional
	Terapista occupazionale
	Tegevusterapeut
	Arbetsterapeut
	Εργοθεραπευτής
	Ergothérapeute
	Ergotherapist
	ерготерапевт
	Stručni prvostupnik/ca radne terapije
	Ergoterapeits
	Ergoterapeutas
	Strukovni radni terapeut
	Tevekenysek terapeuta
	Okupaciuri Terapevti
	Terapeuta Zajęciowy

therapist making it more difficult to give visibility to this profession, as often commissioners, or even patients and clients, do not realize they are benefitting from occupational therapy.

A strong voice for the profession is needed in Europe, acknowledging the three elements of Education, Practice, and Research. This is the reason that COTEC and ENOTHE have worked together, not only to develop a third branch—ROTOS—for Research in Occupational Therapy and Occupational Science, but also to bring together these three bodies, in an umbrella organization called Occupational Therapy Europe, to strengthen the profession Europewide [3]. Occupational Therapy Europe is the umbrella-organization which strives to make the occupational therapy profession visible, valued, available, and accessible for all citizens in Europe.

COTEC is the European organization for all occupational therapists through their National Associations, with the purpose of ensuring an adequate number of high quality occupational therapy practitioners and services in Europe. COTEC is a non-profit organization representing more than 180,000 occupational therapists through the *31 Member Associations*. COTEC is a regional group of the World Federation of Occupational Therapists WFOT. The European Network of Occupational Therapy in Higher Education (ENOTHE) is a non-profit association. The overall concern for the 100 members is with the standards and quality of professional education of occupational therapy across Europe. Research in Occupational Therapy and Occupational Science (ROTOS) is a network organization in development which will unite researchers and support Occupational Therapy Europe and its members with evidence of the (cost) effectiveness of occupational therapy.

This book is important, as we all know ageing and everything that comes with it, is a major issue in the world and in Europe, putting stress on human and financial resources. To tackle these problems, the World Health Organization Regional Office Europe and the European Commission promote a policy of person centered, integrated care (CIHSD) [4–6].

These policies are very much in line with the core principles of Occupational therapy (Table 1.2). And so we, as occupational therapists, should demonstrate we are able to contribute to the solutions to the health and social issues in Europe and find powerful allies to support us and endorse our message. *One of our key messages is not to ask "What is the matter," but rather, "What matters to you?"*

In the current health system, which is very medically and diagnostically driven, the main focus is on "What is the Matter?" [7, 8].

Table 1.2 Core principles of occupational therapy	
	Patient empowerment
	Enabling occupation and participation
	Engaging partnership
	Autonomy and self-management
	Start with the persons wishes on daily occupations
	Quality of life
	Look at the power and possibilities

Diagnosis and treatment is arranged around specialty. When there are multiple diagnoses there are multiple specialists involved. Research and guidelines are organized around diagnosis and disease. So, as an example, a lot is known about how to treat diabetes, or how to treat osteoporosis or depression. However, within an increasingly older population many people have more than one or two chronic disorders, and this means it is difficult to identify what is the effective and right intervention for someone with diabetes, schizophrenia, and COPD—or with osteoporosis, diabetes, and dementia. People with learning disabilities also get older these days, which means issues of empowerment and shared decision-making are a challenge. The real issue being equally concerned with how these co-morbidities impact on a persons' ability to live the life they want to live [7, 8].

The challenges facing healthcare services include an ageing population, and increasing numbers of patients with long-term conditions and multi-morbidities. These populations will benefit from an approach that is focused on persons (rather than patients) and their social network, possibilities, functioning, and quality of life, rather than only on medical treatment of symptoms [7, 8]

The current system is not focused on: "What matters to you?" which means acknowledging the persons wishes, functioning, and quality of life. Although occupational therapists have the medical knowledge, their focus is on the person and his social network, daily functioning, and participation in meaningful occupations and society. Because occupational therapists address the entire area of daily living, they are used to work with other professionals in both health and social care, and also with professionals in the more technical fields, such as architects, ICT, product developers, and designers. This means that occupational therapists are fully equipped to play a central role in primary and integrated care systems [7]. Having an occupational therapist (OT) in a multi-professional team would be helpful in identifying the ways to integrate the health and social services to better effect. Looking for solutions that address the impact of illness or disability, and how individuals participate in society, is the key to robust integrated health care delivery systems [7].

This means we have to take part in interdisciplinary networks where we explain and demonstrate the contribution of occupational therapy. We have to make sure that occupational therapy is seen and acknowledged as a key profession in health and social care. A successful example of a positive and important result of networking and finding influential partners is COTEC's membership of the European Forum of Primary Care (EFPC). The former president of EFPC, Professor Jan de Maeseneer is also the chair of the influential Expert Panel on effective ways of investing in Health (EXPH) that advises the European Commission. In their report "Definition of a frame of reference in relation to Primary Care with special emphasis on financial systems and referral systems" [9] occupational therapy is mentioned as one of the key professions in primary care. It is clear that this opens the possibility of discussing the position of the profession in primary care across Europe.

As OT-Europe is run by volunteers and does not have unlimited resources of workforce or budget, we need to be creative and inclusive in bringing our message to the outside world. That is why COTEC has invested a lot of energy in organizing the occupational therapy community, and in developing external relationships, by signing partnerships, and becoming members of relevant European Networks, e.g., EFPC, EUPHA, Health First Europe, and thematic networks of the Health Policy Platform.

The establishment of the OT-Europe Register of Experts is very important in building a community of occupational therapists, who are able to speak for and about occupational therapy, on a variety of platforms. As occupational therapy has a very broad scope, it is important to identify experts in different fields. The experts are asked to work with COTEC and OT-Europe on a European level, for instance writing position papers, representing the profession in key meetings, and involvement in working groups and thematic networks.

Working in networks is also a mirror of how occupational therapists work in practice.

In daily practice every occupational therapist works in networks which are fitting to and defined by the context of the person who is in need of occupational therapy. As meaningful occupations, context, and daily life are very complicated concepts, even apart from the diagnosis of the person, occupational therapists have to and are used to work with people and professionals not only in health and social care but also in areas like ICT, technology, design, building, education, working conditions service/ safety and health service, and so on. You could even challenge whether an occupational therapist that works alone can deliver high quality all round occupational therapy. Other professionals, like for instance medical consultants often ask occupational therapists: "Why do you make things so complicated, why do you take the whole world into account when you want to make a plan or to make a measurement of behavior?" But taking "the whole world," all aspects of daily life into account is the essential part of the profession and the basis of an occupational perspective of life, as every person is different and unique in his or her wishes, needs, capacities, context, and environment.

Anne Bucher, the Director General of DG Santé, states that more coordination, communication, and inclusiveness are needed to tackle the health issues in Europe. Therefore it is both logic and important that in this book not only occupational therapists are involved, but also psychologists, geriatricians, intensivists (intensive care specialists), elderly specialists (nursing home doctors), psychiatrists, other allied health professionals, welfare professionals, sociologists, designers, and other specialist professions that collaborate to ensure to provide the best care and environment for the ageing population.

The total number of occupational therapists in Europe has increased in the last 5 years with 50,000 to over 180,000 (Fig. 1.1). Becoming a growing and more known profession means that also more students are studying occupational therapy. However, in many countries there is a lack of occupational therapists and students as governments are not convinced yet that occupational therapists can effectively contribute to the health and social issues they are facing.

This book will make a real difference in the field of geriatrics and I am very proud that all the occupational therapy authors in this book are in the Register of

Experts for OT-Europe as experts in their field and are involved in the work of COTEC, making occupational therapy visible, valued, accessible and available for all citizens in Europe.

References

1. COTEC – Council of Occupational Therapists for European Countries [Internet]. [citato 2 aprile 2019]. https://www.coteceurope.eu/.
2. Summary of the Profession – COTEC [Internet]. [citato 2 aprile 2019]. https://www.coteceurope.eu/updates/summary-of-the-profession/.
3. OT EU [Internet]. [citato 2 aprile 2019]. http://www.oteurope.eu/.
4. Health services delivery [Internet]. 2019. [citato 2 aprile 2019]. http://www.euro.who.int/en/health-topics/Health-systems/health-services-delivery/health-services-delivery.
5. Office of the European Union 2017. State of health in the EU companion report 2017 [Internet]. 2017. https://ec.europa.eu/health/sites/health/files/state/docs/2017_companion_en.pdf.
6. Declaration PS. Integrated care [Internet]. Health First Europe. 2017. [citato 2 aprile 2019]. https://healthfirsteurope.eu/topic/european-parliamentary-interest-group-on-innovation-in-health-and-social-care/.
7. Minis M-A, Saenger S, Steultjens E. Occupational therapy perspective on integrated care. Int J Integr Care. 2018;18(s2):265.
8. De Maeseneer J, Boeckxstaens P. James Mackenzie Lecture 2011: multimorbidity, goal-oriented care, and equity. Br J Gen Pract. 2012;62(600):e522–4.
9. Union PO of the E. Definition of a frame of reference in relation to primary care with a special emphasis on financing systems and referral systems. [Internet]. 2015. [citato 2 aprile 2019]. https://publications.europa.eu/en/publication-detail/-/publication/c34869f8-783e-4d99-9f58-6bcd5965608e.

S. Saenger started her career as an occupational therapist in 1978 in Psychiatry where she founded three OT departments and developed OT programs for different client groups. She has been involved in COTEC and ENOTHE since 2000 and was member of the OT Tuning project team. In October 2013 at the first General Assembly of COTEC, Stephanie was elected president of COTEC. In November 2014 she was honored by the Dutch Association with the Astrid Kinébanian Award and in 2017 with the honorary membership.

Team, Occupational Therapist and Geriatrician

Giuseppe Bellelli, Marco Inzitari,
Juan Antonio López Segura, Marie Chantal Morel-Bracq,
and Yann Michel Bertholom

2.1   Introduction and Background

The progressive aging of our society can be depicted as a "silver tsunami" [1], a phenomenon which is rapidly diffusing across all the industrialized countries. Just to put in the context, in 1990, there were 3.1 million US people aged 65 years and older, and in 2005, there were roughly 35.6 [2]. By 2030, according to US estimates, there will be about 71.5 million older persons, more than twice their number in 2000 [3]. Across Organisation for Economic Cooperation and Development (OECD) countries, life expectancy at birth, reached in 2014 on average 80.6 years, an increase of more than 10 years since 1970 [4]. From 1970 to now, life expectancy at

G. Bellelli (✉)
Department of Medicine and Surgery, University of Milano Bicocca, Milan, Italy

Acute Geriatric Unit, San Gerardo Hospital, Monza, Monza, Italy
e-mail: giuseppe.bellelli@unimib.it

M. Inzitari
Parc Sanitari Pere Virgili and Vall d'Hebrón Research Institute, Barcelona, Spain

Universitat Autònoma de Barcelona, Barcelona, Spain

Catalan Society of Geriatrics and Gerontology, Catalonia, Spain
e-mail: minzitari@perevirgili.cat

J. A. L. Segura
Parc Sanitari Pere Virgili and Vall d'Hebrón Research Institute, Barcelona, Spain
e-mail: jlopez@perevirgili.cat

M. C. Morel-Bracq
Directeur des Soins Honoraire, Membre du Comité Scientifique de l'Association Nationale Française des Ergothérapeutes, Bordeaux, France

Y. M. Bertholom
Scientific Board of the Italian Scientific Society of Occupational Therapy, Rome, Italy

Centro Abilitativo del "Paese di Oz" e "Quadrifoglio" di ANFFAS Trento, Trento, Italy

© Springer Nature Switzerland AG 2020
C. Pozzi et al. (eds.), *Occupational Therapy for Older People*,
https://doi.org/10.1007/978-3-030-35731-3_2

birth continues to increase steadily in OECD countries, going up on average by three to four months every year [4]. In this scenario, the "oldest old" are already representing the fastest growing section of elderly population.

The implications of this demographic trend are relevant for healthcare professionals and systems. Over the last decades, the advances in public health and the breakthroughs in medical and surgical sciences have contributed to extend the average life spans of our populations. However, this success in reducing deaths from acute illnesses has resulted in a huge and uncontrolled expansion of chronic diseases. As premature death from acute illness is reduced, the prevalence of conditions that accumulate over time continue to rise and the coexistence of chronic diseases is nowadays the rule rather than exception. Nearly half of Americans have at least one chronic illness accounting for more than three-fourths of America's health care spending [5]. In Italy, according to the National Institute of Statistics, nearly 4 in 10 community-dwellers report having at least one and 2 in 10 report having at least two chronic diseases [6]. Among people aged 75 years and over, 66.7% (58.4% among men and 72.1% among females) are comorbid, i.e., had two or more co-occurring chronic diseases [6]. Furthermore, oldest people are the major users of health-care services and account for more than two-thirds of national health-care costs [7].

Interdisciplinary work is one key approach to the care and management of the older person and of the geriatric patient. The older patients often presents multiple problems and needs, which may include multi-morbidity, geriatric syndromes, cognitive and emotional aspects, frailty, disabilities, lack of social relationships and of social support, and potentially non adapted environments or barriers. Moreover, the management strategies should rely on the own patient values, preferences, and needs, in a shared decision-making approach. Therefore, a multidimensional approach, based on the CGA, and a consequent multi-factorial, individualized treatment plan are warranted, to avoid care fragmentation.

All this management strategy cannot be in charge of a single professional figure, but needs a di-verse expertise pulled together into a team. The Institute of Medicine of the National Academies made a similar plea in the Quality Chasm report, strongly urging that all health professionals receive interdisciplinary team training to ensure the delivery of patient-centered care [8]. The implementation of this interdisciplinary work cannot follow a mere combination of different protocols or processes, but should build on shared goals, tasks, and responsibilities. Organizational aspects, and in particular the interdisciplinary meeting or round, are key to facilitate this approach.

Interdisciplinary teamwork is one of the key elements at the base of the success of different models of geriatric care, starting from acute care [9], to rehabilitation [10] up to community-based care for the frail older person [11].

An occupational therapist is one of the team members involved in the CGA-based model of care. The occupational therapists can plaly multiple tasks within the team. Among all, the assessment of the patient's functional status and ability is one of the most important. It is also important to emphasize the occupational therapist's contribution in assessing, and if necessary, in modifying the physical environment to facilitate the individual's participation. This role is highlighted in the profession's definition, as according to the definition provided by the World Federation of Occupational Therapy [12], occupational therapy is "a client-centred health profession concerned with promoting health and well-being through occupation. The primary goal of occupational therapy is to enable people to participate in the activities of everyday life." This is also consistent with the International Classification of Functioning, Disability and Health (ICF) developed by the WHO [13]. "Occupational therapists achieve this outcome by working with people and communities to enhance their ability to engage in the occupations they want to, need to, or are expected to do, or by modifying the occupation or the environment to better support their occupational engagement" [12].

As can be observed from this definition, the main focus of occupational therapy is "occupation." But what does the word "occupation" exactly mean? The most common understanding of this word in the public feeling concerns an employment (paid or unpaid) or a vocation. However, for the occupational therapists, the term refers to a group of activities and tasks that an individual performs by routine every day, given the values and the meanings of these activities in his/her culture [14]. Occupation is everything people do to occupy themselves, including looking after themselves (self-care), enjoying life (leisure), and contributing to the social and economic fabric of their communities (productivity) [15].

Occupation was the focus of the profession's first paradigm at the beginning of the twentieth century. This paradigm focused on the importance of occupation in human life and health, emphasizing that a lack of occupation could result in damage to the body and mind, and describing its potential use as a therapeutic tool to regenerate the lost function(s). However, in the mid-twentieth century, following the progress of biomedical knowledge and a pressure from the medical world to be rigorous on a scientific perspective, a second paradigm emerged, focusing on the importance of the functioning of various inner systems (neuromotor, musculoskeletal, or intrapsychic functions). It was believed that performance could be improved by addressing these systems; accordingly, the occupational therapy practice changed. An example of translation of these concepts in clinical settings is, for example, the use of decontextualized table top activities (for example, grasp and release exercises or perceptual motor skills retraining). Fortunately, the profession found its way back to occupation. In the 1960s, in the USA, occupational therapy scholars began to call for a new paradigm, focused again on occupation. By the end of the twentieth century, the context acquired greater importance within the health world and the perception of the complexity of disability led to the emergence of a third contemporary paradigm focused on the interaction between the person, occupation, and the environment in a systemic perspective [16].

From this background, it can be seen that occupational therapists have two traditions: one is impairment-based and the other is occupation-based [17]. The Canadian guidelines for occupational therapy practice drew attention to the distinction between these two traditions, arguing that, ultimately, the tradition of occupational therapy must be occupation-based, owing to address impairments only to the extent that they serve occupation [15]. Thus, occupational therapists ought to consider which occupations are important and meaningful to a person, and the ultimate goal should be to improve the individual's participation and engagement in a meaningful occupation [17].

In this chapter we first describe the model of chronic care and integrated care, then we discuss the role of the occupational therapist within the geriatric team, with a detailed description of the main occupation-based practice models.

2.2 The Model of Chronic Care and Integrated Care

2.2.1 A New Paradigm of Care for Older People

In 2004, Tinetti and Fried [18] published a landmark article entitled "The end of the disease era," stating that: "…The time has come to abandon disease as the primary focus of medical care. […] The changed spectrum of health conditions, the complex interplay of biological and non-biological factors, the aging population, and the inter-individual variability in health priorities render medical care that is centered primarily on the diagnosis and treatment of individual diseases at best out-of-date and at worst harmful…" [18]. Why did the authors publish such provocative article? Of course, they did not think that diseases are not important in geriatric clinical practice and that medicine could be stripped of the disease concept; however, they wanted to underscore that a new approach is required to effectively meet the multiple and heterogeneous needs of the majority of older people.

There are at least two reasons explaining why a disease-centered model of care is doomed to fail when applied to an older patient [19]. One of the tenets of the classic medicine is that a treatment should be started only when a diagnosis have been made. In geriatric patients, this tenet may lead to a risk of over-diagnosis, because multiple subclinical and clinical abnormalities are detected simultaneously. With the technology currently available, in fact, we can find pathology wherever we look [20]. An example of the harm caused by overtesting involves measurement of prostate-specific antigen (PSA) to screen for prostate cancer. The introduction of that test has resulted in an epidemic of prostate cancer in older men who otherwise would have lived happily without knowing they had cancer. The quadrupling of the use of radical surgery in these patients is of no proven benefit [21]. Moreover, over-diagnosis may lead to over-treatment. There is a plenty of studies showing that polypharmacy is common in older people and that it is frequently the result of the diagnostic process of multiple conditions. However, many of the drugs which are commonly prescribed in older people have unproven or limited efficacy in these subjects [22].

Paradoxically, a disease-centered model of care may also lead to under- or inappropriate treatment of clinical conditions, due to ageism, poor knowledge of the patient, or lack of evidence-based algorithms applicable to the heterogeneous geriatric population [19]. It is well known that therapeutic algorithms have generally been developed on the basis of evidence resulting from studies carried out in young people, where older people are generally under-represented [23].

In either case, the quality of life of the individual, as well as his/her clinical outcomes, might be substantially and negatively affected. Therefore, the primacy of the diagnosis may lead to a confusion of means with ends [20]. The goal of medicine, on the contrary, is to relieve suffering, to help, and to heal. Correct diagnosis, based on our understanding of pathophysiology, is one means to achieve that goal [20], but is not the aim.

A different and more appropriate approach in geriatric medicine relies on the use of comprehensive geriatric assessment (CGA). This approach has several properties, the most important is that it moves the center of the medical intervention from the individual's disease to his/her overall functioning [19].

The CGA can be defined as a "multidimensional interdisciplinary diagnostic process focused on determining an older person's medical, psychological, and functional capability in order to develop a coordinated and integrated plan for treatment and long-term follow-up [24]. The CGA differs from a standard medical evaluation in that: (a) it assesses also nonmedical domains, including person's functional ability, cognitive status, and socio-environmental condition, as well as an extensive review of prescribed drugs; and (b) it may consider a coordinated multidisciplinary assessment, treatment recommendations made by the multidisciplinary team, and the formation of a plan of care including appropriate rehabilitation and long-term follow-up [25].

The CGA is therefore both a diagnostic and therapeutic process, designed to evaluate all the elements affecting the global health status of an older person. While integrating standard medical diagnostic evaluation, it emphasizes problem-solving and aids in the development of treatment and follow-up plans, in the coordination of management of care and in the evaluation of long-term care needs [25].

The CGA incorporates several domains, each of them containing a number of subdomains, which generally are assessed with the assistance of standardized scales and instruments. Among all assessed within the CGA, the cognitive, functional, and the nutritional domains are key factors.

The incidence of dementia increases with age, particularly among those over 85 years, yet many patients with cognitive impairment remain undiagnosed. The value of making an early diagnosis includes the possibility of uncovering treatable conditions and provides prognostic information that assists in long-term care planning. Cognitive impairment, in fact, is a well-known predictor of negative events, including mortality, institutionalization, disability, and hospitalization [26, 27]. Examples of tools to assess cognitive performances are the Mini Mental State Examination [28] and the Short Portable Status mental Questionnaire [29].

Functional status refers to the ability to perform activities necessary or desirable in daily life. This assessment is particularly important in older people because functional status is directly influenced by health conditions and a sudden change in functional abilities is commonly the presenting symptom of an upcoming acute illness. For example, a sudden imbalance of functional status (e.g., not being able to bathe independently or becoming acutely unable to walk) may be the presenting symptom of pneumonia and acute heart failure [30–32]. Changes in functional status should therefore prompt further diagnostic evaluation and intervention [33].

Additionally, measurement of functional status can be valuable in monitoring response to treatment and can provide prognostic information that assists in long-term care planning. For instance, elevated blood pressure in individuals age 65 and older was associated with increased mortality only in individuals with a walking speed ≥ 0.8 m/s (measured over 6 m or 20 ft.) [34]. Examples of tests to assess functional performances are the short physical performance battery [35] and the activities of daily living (ADL) [36].

The evaluation of nutritional status is also a fundamental part of CGA. Poor nutritional status is common in older people across all settings of care and is frequently the result of changes associated with aging, such as decreases in taste acuity and smell, deteriorating dental health, and decreases in physical activity, which may all affect nutrient intake [37]. As for the cognitive and functional status, addressing patient's nutritional status may be useful not only to plan corrective measures, but also to obtain prognostic information on the risk of medical complications [38] the duration of hospital stay and re-admission to hospital [39, 40].

"Geriatric syndromes" are other particular conditions, which can be best identified using the CGA. "Geriatric syndrome" is a term used to refer to health conditions that do not fit into distinct organ-based disease categories and often have multi-factorial causes. The list includes conditions such as delirium, incontinence, falls, gait disorders, sensory deficits, fatigue, and dizziness. These conditions are common in geriatric care and may have a major impact on survival, disability, cognitive impairment, and the overall quality of life [41–43].

Finally, yet importantly, older patients should also be assessed about the family situation and availability of current caregiver network (if needed), including its deficiencies and potential. Despite frequently neglected, evaluating such domain may have unique implication to optimize the level of care. For instance, assessing the living conditions and the availability of a caregiver to supervise the assumption of prescribed drugs in a person living alone with severe cognitive impairment is crucial to avoid involuntary misassumption and a decompensation of chronic diseases.

2.2.2 The Models of CGA and Geriatric Care

In a Cochrane review published in 2017, Ellis et al summarized the current evidence on CGA effectiveness, comparing its use in older adults after admission to hospital wards with routine care. Among a total population of 13,766 people (29 relevant trials from nine countries), the review showed that patients receiving CGA rather than routine medical care were more likely to be alive and at their home at medium-long-term follow-up [25]. Despite the review did not clarify whether there is a difference in the way the CGA is provided (i.e., whether, for example, it was provided on a specialized geriatric ward or across several wards by a mobile team) [25], this Cochrane definitely supports the need that such approach should become the standard for the assessment and care of older adults admitted to the hospital.

Conceptually, CGA involves several processes that are shared over several professional into the team. The overall care rendered by CGA teams can be divided into six steps: (1) Data-gathering; (2) Discussion among the team, including the patient and/or caregiver as team's member; (3) Development of a treatment plan in accordance with the patient and/or caregiver; (4) Implementation of the treatment plan; (5) Monitoring response to the treatment plan; and (6) Revising the treatment plan.

The range of health care professionals working in the assessment team can vary based on the services provided by individual CGA programs. In many settings, the CGA process relies on a core team including clinician, nurse, and social worker and, when appropriate, draws upon an extended team of physical and occupational therapists, nutritionists, speech therapists, pharmacists, psychologists, podiatrists, and others. Traditionally, the geriatrician evaluates a list of medical conditions and provides initial assessments or screening for specific CGA domains. On its side, the nurse evaluates other domains, including the risk of fall and of developing pressure sores, and the level of assistance required to guarantee the patient's safety during hospital admission. This information should be subsequently augmented with more in-depth evaluations by additional professionals. As an example, a physical therapist can evaluate the patient's impairment in gait and balance, an occupational therapist may be needed to conduct a more extensive assessment on patient's independence in self-caring and a nutritionist to evaluate the need for specific nutritional support.

2.2.3 Delivering Integrated Care to Patients with Chronic Diseases

There is no unifying definition or common conceptual understanding of integrated care [44], but, generally, it is defined in contrast to fragmented and episodic care.

There are at least two reasons why integrated care is better than fragmented care when the subject of intervention is an older subject. Acute diseases are profoundly different from chronic diseases (Table 2.1).

For instance, acute diseases are usually isolated to one bodily area and respond to treatment, whereas, in contrast, chronic diseases frequently involve multiple systems, have a future characterized by fluctuations between relapses and remissions. Additionally, full recovery or healing is a peculiarity of acute diseases but it is not possible in chronic diseases. This means that suffering from multiple chronic diseases implies the patients could be able to deal with his/her own illness for the rest of the life. To support this statement, Hopman and colleagues [45] showed that people with multi-morbidity vary greatly regarding their needs for care and support: many of them have problems and in different domains of life, which may ask for more extensive care and support (e.g., including mental health care, social care, or community services), and interdisciplinary approach. Therefore, whereas acute diseases can be successfully treated with a series of interventions not necessarily factored in a coordinated manner, chronic diseases necessarily require a connection of these interventions.

Table 2.1 Differences between acute and chronic diseases

	Acute disease	Chronic disease
Definition	An acute disease is a disease with a rapid onset and/or a short course	A chronic disease is a disease that is persistent or otherwise long-lasting in its effects. The term chronic is usually applied when the course of the disease lasts for more than 3 months
Appearance of symptoms	Sudden	Usually gradual
Duration	Short; a few days to a week or 2 weeks	Extended period of time; usually 6 weeks or more, often months or years
Treatment	Some acute diseases (e.g., influenza) can be resolved without treatment. Other acute diseases, like pneumonia, may require anything from over-the-counter or prescription drugs to hospital care	Chronic diseases cannot be cured, but treatment may alleviate the symptoms. Periodically chronic diseases may require hospitalization. In general, chronic diseases require multiple inputs from several professionals working in the same team (multidisciplinary approach) at a hospital ward
Prolonged care	Not needed, generally	An extended period of care after hospitalization and an integration among professionals is mandatory. Patients with chronic diseases benefit highly from supportive networks with people who understand their struggles
Examples	Bone fracture, flu, pneumonia, asthma attack, heartburn	Osteoporosis, heart failure, kidney disease, Alzheimer's disease and dementia, diabetes

The integrated care model for patients with chronic disease requires a standardized method to be delivered. The methods and the organizational aspects to deliver such model of care will be discussed in the following section of this chapter. What is very important is that this model of care is effective in improving the quality of assistance and in reducing mortality of patients with chronic diseases who receive it [46]. This kind of approach can also result in greater patient satisfaction with the treatment, in a reduction of the average length of hospital stay and of unplanned hospital readmissions [47, 48]. Recently, a quasi-experimental longitudinal study compared the clinical impact of a home-based Intermediate care model in the Catalan health system with a usual bed-based care [49]. A total of 849 subjects (244 in the Hospital-at-Home Unit and 605 in the bed-based Intermediate Care unit, mean age 83.2 years) were included. The home-based scheme showed better results on functional resolution, on favorable crisis resolution, and on the length of intervention, which was globally shorter than for usual care. Importantly, hospital-at-home model in this study extended the CGA-based intervention to the rehabilitation phase, tailoring the intervention to the "whole" (clinical and functional) resolution of the health crisis, indirectly suggesting that multidisciplinary patient-centered care plans using a flexible approach to deliver care might are really effective to meet the older patient's needs [49].

2.3   The Occupational Therapist Within the Geriatric Team

2.3.1   What Is a Team?

The Health Care Team Effectiveness Project, NHS [5] defines a team as "a group of individuals with different roles that work together to produce products" or, in the case of healthcare, "to deliver services for which they are mutually accountable. Team members share goals and are mutually held accountable for meeting them, they are inter-dependent in their accomplishment and they affect the results through their interaction with one another. Because the team is held collectively accountable, the work of integrating with one another is included among responsibilities of each member."

In the following paragraphs, we will review the ideal functioning and key elements of success of teamwork in geriatrics, including aspects pertaining to the organization and to the workforce and its management (Table 2.2). As a bottom line, high performing teams and a well-functioning teamwork have shown to improve the results in terms of quality of patients care while innovating in care provision and delivery, with lower levels of stress [50]. In 1995, The American Geriatrics Society developed a position statement on interdisciplinary care for older adults, which supports the interdisciplinary care model for the following reasons [51]:

1. Interdisciplinary care meets the complex needs of older adults with multiple, inter-acting comorbidities.
2. Interdisciplinary care improves health care processes and outcomes for geriatric syndromes.
3. Interdisciplinary care benefits the health care system as well as caregivers of older adults.
4. Interdisciplinary training and education effectively prepares providers to care for older adults.

Table 2.2 Elements supporting the need of interdisciplinary teamwork as a pillar, in geriatrics

Problems/needs	Recommended approach
Multiple problems and needs (including medical aspects, geriatric syndromes, functional, mental, and social-environmental aspects)	Comprehensive geriatric assessment (CGA), need of complementary expertise and management of care transitions
Fluctuating and dynamic clinical and functional course	Dynamic view (which is the recent evolution?) and prognosis
Social and economic needs	Adequate management of the available resources
Need of a holistic bio-psycho-social approach	Shared decision-making, taking into account patients goals, values, and preferences
Uncertainty in the application of evidence-based approaches and in the definition of the prognosis	Contextualization and interpretation of the available evidence

2.3.2 Organizational Aspects: How Interdisciplinary Meetings Should Work

Interdisciplinary teamwork dynamics are well established in geriatrics, and different reports and gray papers have summarized possible aspects to implement its successful routine functioning (Table 2.3).

A key point for a smooth, effective, and efficient teamwork is a formal meeting, which could be defined as "interdisciplinary round." This meeting needs a fixed schedule and an agenda in the routine work, either in the acute or post-acute hospital ward, in the community or in a nursing home. Frequency is variable depending on the specific resource: for example, in an acute ward or in palliative care, where the care episode is shorter and the turnover is higher, a daily meeting is warranted, with an additional weekly meeting reserved for the most complex cases, those characterized by uncertainty of the prognosis or special management difficulties. Conversely, in a post-acute environment, weekly meetings are preferred, and in a community or nursing home settings, although a weekly meeting dynamic can be organized, each individual patient's evolution and care plan can be revised at fixed schedules, for example, each month or 3–6 months, with flexibility in case of sudden changes in their health or social status. As for the specific dynamic or protocol to put in place during the meeting, it needs a certain degree of contextualization, depending on the functioning, roles, and level of maturity of the team. However, a contextualized specific protocol is recommended, to guarantee an effective and efficient work [52]. Depending on the setting, the leadership can be attributed to the physician (usually in acute setting) or nurses (usually in long-term facilities or nursing homes) with a range of "gray zones" in the middle, where different leaderships can be assigned depending on the individual figures. The leader acts as a moderator and might help to disentangle conflicts or situations with contrasting viewpoints, preferably through the discussion. As for each member's specific contribution, the physician updates the team on the clinical aspects (medical history, examination, etc.), including the assessment of frailty plus the medication review; the nurse adds on the functional status (with updated quantitative measures), vital signs, geriatric syndromes, such as pain control, nutrition and hydration, elimination (urine and bowel), mobility, delirium,

Table 2.3 Steps of the interdisciplinary meeting

Plan the meeting using agendas
Define roles (moderator/leader, secretary)
Establish a round for sharing information based on each profession's specificity, based on a bio-psycho-social view
Follow-up on the patient's evolution (also using quantitative tools)
Define patient's goals, preferences, and values
Define and list problems and needs
Design a tailored approach
Define the follow-up, and, in case, the discharge plan
Share the plan with the patient (and the caregiver if needed)
Leave a clear and visible track of the agreements and plan on the patient's health records

and also on quality and safety aspects (catheters, IV lines, pressure ulcers, falls, infection control, etc.); the physical therapist adds specific information on mobility and the physical status, orienting the plan for rehabilitation, exercise, and physical activity, and the social worker on social aspects and the activation of social resources. Regarding the role of the occupational therapist, we devote a specific paragraph on this specific role in the team, but generally, he/she might add specific information on functional status and cognitive aspects, also with recommendations for the care plan, from a patient-centered perspective, and also focuses on the environment and on support products. Regarding the other professionals (psychologist or neuropsychologist, pharmacist, etc.) each would add information about their specific assessments.

A key actor in the interdisciplinary round is the patient, and, in case, the caregiver. The patient's goals, preferences, and values are pivotal to establish the individualized care plan, and the ideal scenario is that the patient and, in case the patient agrees, the caregiver, are included in the meeting. Although in the "real life," for efficiency reasons, the constant physical participation of patients in the meeting, mainly in cases of frail persons with cognitive impairment, might result a very complex task, the effort of the teams, institutions and systems should be oriented towards that model. On the other side, in case the patients, in environments with a higher turnover and shorter stays, cannot be systematically involved in the meetings, specific sessions dedicated to this shared goals and direct feedback work should be planned. In any case, after the meetings, in case the person and caregivers are not directly involved, a feedback with them should be maintained, at least by a designated team representative or by the team leader: information about the evolution, goals, care plan, and discharge arrangements should be provided in a plain language and allowing an open discussion, and the patient should be prompted to express his/her doubts and concerns.

The final goal of the meeting depends on the stage for the care episode: (1) in the first meeting the goal will be to agree upon a global dynamic picture of the patient, meaning that the retrospective reconstruction of the clinical and functional evolution which brought to the current status is key for the prognosis and the care plan; this picture is based on the CGA, with the contribution of the whole team. The main problems and needs of the person will be listed, in a clear way which will allow an easy follow-up. In this meeting, shared goals, with a short- and long-term perspective, will be set, and an individualized care plan will be designed; (2) in the follow-up meetings, the evolution of the clinical and functional status, also supported by the re-assessment through quantitative scales, is warranted, with consequent adjustments in the care plan; (3) in case of hospitalized patients, a discharge date and a discharge plan including continuity of care aspects will be discussed and set; (4) in the final meeting, all this plan will be confirmed.

Each meeting should be "wrapped-up" and summarized in the patient's health record, as a formal reference for the team members, other professionals who could not join the meeting, and for the follow-up. The notes should include schematic information about problems/needs, summary evolution, also quantified by functional scales, shared short- and long-term goals, the main actions of the individualized care plan and the discharge arrangements, when adequate.

2.3.3   Workforce and Talent: The Successful Team

Organizational aspects and the institutional culture are relevant, but, as many other activities carried out by persons, the success of teamwork depends on the contribution of its members, which is largely based on the personal skills, knowledge and training, traits and motivations, or, in other words, on the individual talent. Not all the team members have to contribute in the same way, and in fact, roles are an important aspect of teamwork. However, teams with a higher proportion of individuals with talent for the teamwork have a higher performance.

The talent for teamwork is the resultant of a mix of: (1) skills, such as leadership, negotiation, conflict management, ability to listen and influence, decision-making, orientation to evaluation, self- and team management and efficiency, verbal and written communication, and ability to give feedback; (2) knowledge, including aspects of geriatric care, case/care management, organizational goals and strategies, team process; (3) traits, including inter-personal relations, respect for others, cooperative attitude, assertive behavior, self-confidence, toleration to stress, sense of humor; (4) motivation, including commitment to patient care, quality outcome, organization and to work collaboratively [53]. All this skill mix goes beyond the training of one discipline, and training curricula of the implicated healthcare professions should incorporate these skills and training.

In a team, one or more leaders act as catalyzers of the work, and one designated leading role is warranted. Although different leadership styles can be pursued or promoted, also depending on the organizational culture, the tasks required to a modern leader include clarity, delegation, and organization, support to the team and defense and potentiation of its members, feedback and recognition, commitment of pursuing shared decision-making. Integrity and ethical principles, as well as organizational capacities and an appropriate mix of the above mentioned characteristics, are required to work in institutions where teamwork is key. In general, leadership by geriatricians has shown to contribute to high performance care models for older adults with complex needs [54], but also occupational therapists, who sum up technical skills for care and rehabilitation of persons with complex needs with a multi-factorial and pragmatic view, oriented to problem-solving to meet functional goals within a real environment, might represent ideal leading figures in certain settings with a lower patients turnover.

On the other hand, although the individual members and the talent contribute to an important proportion of the successful teamwork, facilitating elements which should be provided from an institutional level, include the clear indication of goals and processes and the support of information technology (well design health electronic records which facilitate information sharing and goals setting and review).

2.3.4   Team Dysfunctions and Cycles in Time

The general theory of teamwork, translated from business models, indicates that different elements of the team constitutions can explain why some teams do not work [55]. These include:

1. Lack of heterogeneity in team expertise and attitudes (constructive criticism and thinking "out of the box" by some team members helps)
2. Teams with an excessive number of members (more than 10)
3. Lack of clarity in the goals
4. Lack of defined functional aspects (periodic interdisciplinary meeting, spaces for exchange and team building)
5. Excessive turnover of team members

Since it is based on a group of individuals, teams experience phases, also in the healthcare or clinical environment. According to a classical scheme which can be also applied to this specific case (Tuckman diagram) [56], standard phases include a "forming" or initial phase, usually characterized by enthusiasm and optimism, but also by anticipation and anxiety, followed by a "storming" phase, characterized by frustration caused by the experience of divergences and dysfunction in the day by day. If the team was well built and is supported and empowered, a "norming" phase follows, characterized by a progressive organization and cohesion, through shared goals, coping and acceptance of individual differences. In the best cases, this phase can be followed by a "performing" phase, with cohesiveness and clear leadership, and the results, in terms of patients' care and members' motivation, are clearly improved. However, "adjourning" phases, marked by tiredness, dissatisfaction, and anxiety, have to be foreseen and possibly anticipated, reviewing the team functioning and also its composition, if possible. Crises might be seen as opportunities to review the teamwork and improve it.

2.3.5   Teamwork Within Integrated Care

If interdisciplinary and teamwork is one of the bases of geriatrics, different types of teams may be needed for the care of the older person, according to the context and to patients' needs. The basic team is obviously the interdisciplinary team that takes care of the patient in the ward or in the community. However, the multiple needs of the older patient often drive that different specialized profiles from different care levels might be required for a shorter and more intensive or prolonged time, to take care of the person during a care transition or a crisis. This might happen more often in the community, where an integrated approach between primary care, which guarantees the care continuum, playing as a "pivot" in the care for the older persons with complex needs, plus specialized geriatric care and social services might be required to act as a functional team, with a smooth coordination. Sometimes, other specialists need to be involved. Therefore, "parallel" or "functional" teams might be necessary for the care of older persons with complex needs, or during specific crises. It is straightforward that these situations of functional coordination or integration are even more challenging compared to the usual teamwork, where a single team is in charge of the patient [57]. In this sense, a real "integrated care" framework requires stable mechanisms and dynamics of functional coordination between levels of care or between different institutions, and/or between health and social care, with predefined protocols or clinical pathways, and hopefully established roles. This scenario is the most suitable for the care of the older person, for their frequent coexisting health, social, and functional needs [13].

Theoretically, it can be reached through macro-integration (a single provider taking care of a whole population or area, and determining the rules of coordination and integration), meso-integration (a single provider or resource taking care of a group of persons with higher needs, such as vulnerable or frail older persons), or micro-integration (utilization of multiple micro-strategies of coordination, including, for example, liaison figures, such as care managers, interdisciplinary meetings between the different teams, shared health electronic records, telemedicine, shared financial incentives, etc.). The experiences that provided the most promising results are mainly oriented to meso-integration (such as the PACE model to maintain home older adults with criteria for institutionalization, or other integrated care model for older adults such as GRACE) [58]. Looking at the impact on the health and well-being of older adults, less evidence exist at macro- and micro-integration levels (quote in case), in part for the challenges and limitations in measuring the impact of such complex interventions through well-designed studies in relatively heterogeneous populations and short follow-up times.

2.3.6 Role of the Occupational Therapist Within the Team

Occupational therapists typically work as team members, providing occupational therapy-specific services, case management, program coordination, and management in the geriatric setting. The main characteristics and added values of these professionals within the team are: (1) the patient-centered approach and the partnership with patients and caregivers, which is intrinsically part of the occupational therapists profession; (2) the understanding of the functional abilities and occupation as the results of the interaction between the intrinsic capacity and the environment [59]. Specific contributions of occupational therapists mainly include the functional assessment [60] and skill development. However, the role of occupational therapists is not limited to skills training, but has a participatory and action-based orientation. As major components of this work, they facilitate direct experiences of engaging in real occupations, either at an individual or group level, and processes that foster autonomy of the person in terms of decision-making and problem-solving [59]. They also work on the assessment and modification of the environment [61], contribute to identify community resources to give support to patients' needs, together with other figures, such as social workers. As a base for this work, occupational therapists evaluate and understand how "ordinary" occupations might be meaningful and contribute to the reablement or well-being of the users. In case of older persons, often these activities are related to the history of occupation (previous work or leisure time activities), together with the current, daily life activities.

Occupational therapists are committed to participation in interdisciplinary teams, and value practice based on partnerships. Occupational therapists gather occupational histories, including information about patient' past and present occupations, interests, skills, community resources, and supports, as a basis to design interdisciplinary care and treatment plans. Occupational therapists also evaluate real life task performance related to specific daily life occupations (e.g., of self-care, home care, work, etc.), with a particular expertise and emphasis regarding the more meaningful ones for the person. In this sense, tools such as the Canadian Occupational Performance Measure© [62], are useful to assess the person-center level of independence in daily life, overcoming potential biases of other functional scales which do not take into account the occupational history of that person [14]. Finally, they take care of the assessment of specific functional deficits, such as the cognitive ones, and of the specific individualized occupational-based plans to reinforce those areas, in collaboration with other disciplines, such as neuropsychology. This is specifically relevant because it is related with personal autonomy and a person-centered approach.

A document by the College for Occupational Therapists of UK focused on the value of this profession to reduce the pressure on hospitals recommends all the rapid response crisis and emergency teams to include occupational therapists, as well as the frailty and rehabilitation teams [63]. The participation of the occupational therapists in these teams improves the performance, for example, reducing hospital admissions. On the other hand, according to the same work, occupational therapists have to be part of the discharge teams.

In summary, specific contributions of the occupational therapists to the interdisciplinary teamwork include:

1. Assessment and identification of the main areas and components of the occupational history—past and present—of the person, with a specific emphasis of the meaningful activities.
2. Implementation of a tailored plan to train, compensate or adapt the deficits aimed to regain the maximum independence in daily life
3. Assessment and intervention on the environment, in order to improve accessibility, functional independence, and security
4. Assessment and recommendation on ergonomic strategies and the use of support products
5. Assessment and training of cognitive function
6. Within the discharge plan, identification of the available support resources
7. Involvement and training for the caregivers

2.4 Main Occupation-Based Practice Models

2.4.1 Two Internationally Recognized Occupational Therapy Conceptual Models: The Model of Human Occupation (MOHO) and the Canadian Model of Occupational Performance and Engagement (CMOP-E)

These models were developed in order to fit the contemporary paradigm of occupational therapy [16], focused on occupation within a complex interaction between the person, the occupation, and the environment. They are built upon a rigorous scientific research, with a humanistic approach, are client-centered, and focus on occupational engagement. These models offer clear guidelines and assessment tools to occupational therapists in a wide range of practice domains, especially in complex domains such as the geriatric practice [16, 64].

2.4.2   Model of Human Occupation (MOHO)

The model of human occupation (MOHO) was first developed during the 1980s by Kielhofner and Burke [65]. The objective of the model is to explain the dynamic and complex interactions of human engagement in occupation, through the person's motivation and capacities, the demand of the task, and the environment opportunities. In occupational therapy, the interventions aim to help clients to adapt and participate in their own environment, focused on the person's singularity [66, 67]. According to this view [67, 68], occupational participation (i.e., the person's engagement in daily living occupations given a specific context) is the result of a dynamic interaction between volition, habituation, and performance capacity within the environment. One of the central concepts, volition, is placing actions, thoughts, and feelings as the core dynamic of therapy. Volition refers to the motivation for occupation and is underpinned by interests, values, and personal causation referring to one's sense of capacity and effectiveness. Another central concept, habituation, refers to the process by which occupation is organized into patterns or routines [67]. Habits and roles are internalized as we grow and act in our own environment. They make daily occupations easy to perform and give us a feeling of familiarity. A third central concept, performance capacity, refers to the physical and mental abilities that underlie skilled occupational performance [67]. Occupational performance is realized through motor skills, process skills, and communication and interaction skills. Performance capacity is strongly linked with the subjective experience, referred to as the lived body [67].

Many assessment tools have been developed consistent with this model. Two of them are widely used in occupational therapy and will be briefly presented here: the Model of Human Occupation Screening Tool (MOHOST) [65] and the Assessment of Motor and Process Skills (AMPS) [69, 70]. The MOHOST provides information at a glance of the person's occupational participation [65]. It explores the person's occupational functioning according to the main MOHO concepts: motivation for occupation (volition), pattern of occupation (habituation), communication and interaction skills, process skills, motor skills (performance capacity), and the environment. Information is gained through observation and informal interviews. Each item is scored in a similar way. In detail, motivation for occupation is evaluated according to the person's appraisal of ability, expectation of success, interest, and choices, while the pattern of occupation is evaluated according to the person's adaptability, roles, and responsibility. Communication and interaction skills include non-verbal skills, conversation, vocal expression, and relationships, whereas process skills include knowledge, timing, organization, and problem-solving, motor skills include posture and mobility, coordination, strength and effort, and energy. Finally, the environment in which the assessment is performed is evaluated for how easy it is to move across the physical space, given the physical resources, the social groups, and the occupational demands [65].

The evaluations allow the occupational therapist to measure the person's strengths and limitations for his/her participation in daily life. Each evaluation is client-centered, occupation focused and takes in account the physical and human environment in its complexity. As much of the required information is based on observation, this assessment is appropriate for elderly people, even with cognitive impairments [65].

The second assessment, the AMPS [70], is complementary to the MOHOST. It focuses on the quality of occupational performance, specifically the motor and process skills, and can be used as an objective measure of change in ADL performance. The AMPS includes more than 140 standardized ADL tasks, ranging in complexity from simple to complex.

Compared to many impairment-focused assessments, the AMPS is based on a top-down approach. This means that it does not test the body function but the quality of occupational performance. The occupational therapist observes the person who is performing two specific tasks, selected in accordance with the person's attitude and capacities to perform them, [70] and rates 16 motor skills, such as body position (stabilizes, aligns, etc.), holding objects (coordinates, manipulates, etc.), sustaining performance (endures, paces, etc.), as well ADL process skills, such as applying knowledge (chooses, notices, etc.) or organizing space and objects (gathers, organizes, etc.), and so on. Each item is rated on a four-point ordinal scale. The AMPS may be used even with older individuals, including low functioning clients, and it is a good predictor of occupational performance at home after hospital discharge [70, 71].

2.4.3 Canadian Model of Occupational Performance and Engagement (CMOP-E)

The Canadian Model of Occupational Performance (CMOP) was proposed in Canada several years after the MOHO, in order to define occupational therapy in the Canadian health system. Occupation was reported as fundamental in occupational therapy and described as a human need. Occupational therapists use the therapeutic potential of occupation to help clients maintain or consolidate their health. A strong humanistic approach encourages a real client-centered intervention towards significant objectives negotiated together. It was a real shift from impairment-focused objectives towards occupational objectives [15]. This model subsequently evolved to place further emphasis on the importance of engagement, being renamed the Canadian model of occupational performance and engagement (CMOP-E) [64].

The CMOP-E describes the person as having physical, affective, cognitive components along with spirituality. It also describes three main categories of occupation: self-care, productivity, and leisure, within the physical, social, institutional, and cultural environment. The interaction between the person, occupation, and environment is termed occupational performance. The CMOP-E relies on occupational science research to better understand occupation and occupational engagement [64]. Enabling occupation is consistent with the ICF standard [13] as based on the social and medical conditions. The social participation is crucial. Therefore, occupational justice is a central concept in the model [64].

An assessment tool has been developed in line with this model: the Canadian occupational performance measure (COPM). The COPM is an occupation-based, client-centered, evidence-based outcome measure used during the assessment process in order to identify the important daily occupations that are restricted by health problems in the areas of self-care, productivity, and leisure. The individual will first provide a list of problems in carrying out an occupational performance, that is a list of the significant occupations that he/she wants to, needs to, or is expected to do, but he/she cannot do, does not do or is not satisfied with the way he/she performs them. Thereafter, the person selects the five most important or pressing occupations and scores them on a scale from 1 to 10 with regard to performance and satisfaction. Thus, the person is asked to rate both the way he/she currently performs the occupation and the level of satisfaction with how he/she performs the occupation. These occupations are then transformed into occupational therapy objectives. Therefore, these significant activities or occupations can be used as a way to develop skills but also as the objective of the rehabilitation process. At the end of the intervention, the rating by the individual will be asked again and the change in performance and satisfaction will serve as an outcome of the therapeutic process [72].

A recent review shows that the COPM has an impact on the clients' awareness of their own needs, therefore improving their motivation [73]. It also represents a good method to make evident the most significant occupations among older people [74] and to facilitate the collaboration between the occupational therapist and the older adult when negotiating the therapeutic objectives. Interview competencies are required from the occupational therapist and also a clear understanding of the power of occupation as it uses a top-down approach. When working in a medical context, occupational therapists can find the COPM use difficult as the objectives are often linked to the clients' occupational performance in their own environment. This is why van Seben et al. recommended further research on its psychometric properties before it is grated as a strong goal-setting instrument in geriatric rehabilitation [75].

Overall, these occupational therapy assessments (MOHOST, AMPS, and COPM) seem globally consistent with the ICF principles, which is useful when working in a team, as it facilitates the communication and the collaboration with other health care professionals [76].

2.4.4 Evolution of Occupational Therapy Practice

Consistent with the evolution of the health system at a global level, moving from cure to care, highlighting prevention, occupational therapists are now increasingly working with frail older people living at home and with their carers to prevent institutionalization. A practice model used with people with Alzheimer's disease and their carers is the community occupational therapy in dementia (COTID). COTID proposes an evidence-based program aiming to help individuals with mild to moderate dementia and their carers living at home to improve daily functioning and reduce the carer's burden. This practice model stands upon MOHO with a systemic perspective [77, 78].

However, occupational science is now informing occupational therapy by producing evidence-based practice and knowledge on occupation and on the way to improve people lives [79]. A promising prevention program is the Lifestyle Redesign® developed by Florence Clark in the USA with elderly clients living at home: the Well Elderly Studies [80, 81]. It is a prevention treatment approach developed by occupational therapists to help older clients improve their health and well-being, by changing their lifestyle to a more healthier routine and occupational balance. The Lifestyle Redesign® is manualized and can be used by trained occupational therapists [82].

2.5 Conclusion

The progressive aging of the population imposes new challenges for the healthcare professionals working with older people. Traditional approaches focusing on the disease as the core of medical intervention should be replaced by new approaches using CGA as the preferred method to assess the various needs of older people and face them. CGA is provided by multidisciplinary professionals to assess the various bio-psycho-social domains and get the patient the appropriate care in a coordinated manner. The benefit of such approach has been clearly demonstrated in studies and meta-analysis, reporting positive outcomes for the patients and satisfaction for caregivers. A progressive implementation of CGA in the routine clinical practice is urgently required for a better healthcare of the older people.

Interdisciplinary teamwork is a key in geriatric care, and organizational aspects and specific skills are needed. Within integrated care models between different care levels or between health and social services, this teamwork might be also needed and is particularly challenging. The contribution of the occupational therapist is central, because it adds relevant and differential aspects, which represent a real value for the teamwork and for the individualized approach to the older persons.

Occupational therapy conceptual models and occupational science have brought a change of perspective leading to client-centered and occupation-based occupational therapy. The pragmatic use in clinical practice of an occupational therapy conceptual model and its associated tools of assessment allows us to more effectively focus on the various aspects of our profession and capture its uniqueness. The information we can gather allow us to trace the occupational therapy process, gather a better occupational understanding of the person and personalize an intervention plan. Occupation is the core of occupational therapy and a health determinant that is now recognized by the team in geriatric care.

Summary with Key Messages

1. In an aging population, older adults often have multi-factorial problems and needs, which require an interdisciplinary alliance and teamwork.
2. Comprehensive geriatric approach (CGA) is an effective multidimensional approach to evaluate the patient's bio-psycho-social domains. It differs from a standard medical evaluation because it assesses also nonmedical domains

(i.e., person's functional ability, cognitive status, and socio-environmental condition as well as a review of prescribed drugs) and involves the participation of several health professionals, which work in a coordinated and complementary manner.

3. The occupational therapist plays a pivotal role in a geriatric team, because it brings differential information on functional and environmental aspects, and participates in the design and implementation of the individualized treatment plan, through a patient participatory approach and by training skills and educating the patient and the caregiver.

4. Organizational aspects, such as a well-structured and directed interdisciplinary round or meeting, are basic for an optimal teamwork.

5. A progressive implementation of CGA in the routine clinical practice as a method to diagnose and treat the multiple unmet needs of older people is urgently required for a better healthcare.

References

1. Fox S. Older Americans and the internet. Washington: Pew Internet and American Life Project; 2004.
2. American Geriatrics Society (AGS), Association of Directors of Geriatric Academic Programs (ADGAP). Geriatric medicine: a clinical imperative for an aging population, part I. Ann Long-Term Care. 2005;13(3):18–22.
3. Tinetti ME, Fried TR, Boyd CM. Designing health care for the most common chronic condition--multimorbidity. JAMA. 2012;307(23):2493–4.
4. OECD. Society at a Glance 2016: OECD Social Indicators. Paris: OECD Publishing; 2016.
5. Ward BW, Schiller JS, Goodman RA. Multiple chronic conditions among US adults: a 2012 update. Prev Chronic Dis. 2014;11:E62.
6. Sistema statistico nazionale Istituto nazionale di statistica. Annuario Statistico Italiano. Roma: ISTAT; 2017. www.istat.it. ISBN 978-88-458-1932-2.
7. Salute Md. Rapporto sull'attività di ricovero ospedaliero. Dati SDO 2016; 2017.
8. Institute of Medicine. Crossing the quality chasm: a new health system for the 21st century; 2001. http://www.nap.edu/books/0309072808/html/.
9. Baztan JJ, Suarez-Garcia FM, Lopez-Arrieta J, Rodriguez-Manas L, Rodriguez-Artalejo F. Effectiveness of acute geriatric units on functional decline, living at home, and case fatality among older patients admitted to hospital for acute medical disorders: meta-analysis. BMJ. 2009;338:b50.
10. Bachmann S, Finger C, Huss A, Egger M, Stuck AE, Clough-Gorr KM. Inpatient rehabilitation specifically designed for geriatric patients: systematic review and meta-analysis of randomised controlled trials. BMJ. 2010;340:c1718.
11. Beswick AD, Rees K, Dieppe P, Ayis S, Gooberman-Hill R, Horwood J, et al. Complex interventions to improve physical function and maintain independent living in elderly people: a systematic review and meta-analysis. Lancet. 2008;371(9614):725–35.
12. World Federation of Occupational Therapists. Definition of occupational therapy; 2012. http://www.wfot.org/.
13. World Health Organization. International statistical classification of diseases and related health problems. 10th revision. Geneva: World Health Organization; 2001. https://www.who.int/classifications/icd/ICD10Volume2_en_2010.pdf.

14. Thyer L, Brown T, Roe D. The Validity of the Canadian Occupational Performance Measure (COPM) when used in a sub-acute rehabilitation setting with older adults. Occup Ther Health Care. 2018;32(2):137–53.
15. Canadian Association of Occupational Therapists. Occupational therapy guidelines for client-centred practice. Toronto; 1991.
16. Kielhofner G. Conceptual foundations of occupational therapy. 4th ed. Philadelphia: F.A. Davis; 2009.
17. Ianes P, Polatajko H. L'enablement dell'occupazione: una prospettiva centrata sul cliente, basata sull'occupazione e orientate al miglioramento della vita. G Ital Ter Occup. 2010;5:49–64.
18. Tinetti ME, Fried T. The end of the disease era. Am J Med. 2004;116(3):179–85.
19. Cesari M, Marzetti E, Thiem U, Pérez-Zepeda MU, Abellan Van Kan G, Landi F, et al. The geriatric management of frailty as paradigm of "The end of the disease era". Eur J Intern Med. 2016;31:11–4.
20. Goodwin JS. Geriatrics and the limits of modern medicine. N Engl J Med. 1999;340(16):1283–5.
21. Johansson JE, Holmberg L, Johansson S, Bergström R, Adami HO. Fifteen-year survival in prostate cancer. A prospective, population-based study in Sweden. JAMA. 1997;277(6):467–71.
22. Brath H, Mehta N, Savage RD, Gill SS, Wu W, Bronskill SE, et al. What is known about preventing, detecting, and reversing prescribing cascades: a scoping review. J Am Geriatr Soc. 2018;66(11):2079–85.
23. Cherubini A, Del Signore S, Ouslander J, Semla T, Michel JP. Fighting against age discrimination in clinical trials. J Am Geriatr Soc. 2010;58(9):1791–6.
24. Rubenstein LZ, Stuck AE, Siu AL, Wieland D. Impacts of geriatric evaluation and management programs on defined outcomes: overview of the evidence. J Am Geriatr Soc. 1991; 39(9 Pt 2):8S. 16S; discussion 7S-8S.
25. Ellis G, Gardner M, Tsiachristas A, Langhorne P, Burke O, Harwood RH, et al. Comprehensive geriatric assessment for older adults admitted to hospital. Cochrane Database Syst Rev. 2017;9:CD006211.
26. Connors MH, Sachdev PS, Kochan NA, Xu J, Draper B, Brodaty H. Cognition and mortality in older people: the Sydney Memory and Ageing Study. Age Ageing. 2015;44(6):1049–54.
27. Zekry D, Herrmann FR, Grandjean R, Vitale AM, De Pinho MF, Michel JP, et al. Does dementia predict adverse hospitalization outcomes? A prospective study in aged inpatients. Int J Geriatr Psychiatry. 2009;24(3):283–91.
28. Folstein MF, Folstein SE, McHugh PR. "Mini-mental state". A practical method for grading the cognitive state of patients for the clinician. J Psychiatr Res. 1975;12(3):189–98.
29. Pfeiffer E. A short portable mental status questionnaire for the assessment of organic brain deficit in elderly patients. J Am Geriatr Soc. 1975;23(10):433–41.
30. Bellelli G, Speciale S, Morghen S, Torpilliesi T, Turco R, Trabucchi M. Are fluctuations in motor performance a diagnostic sign of delirium? J Am Med Dir Assoc. 2011;12(8):578–83.
31. Berman P, Hogan DB, Fox RA. The atypical presentation of infection in old age. Age Ageing. 1987;16(4):201–7.
32. Grosmaitre P, Le Vavasseur O, Yachouh E, Courtial Y, Jacob X, Meyran S, et al. Significance of atypical symptoms for the diagnosis and management of myocardial infarction in elderly patients admitted to emergency departments. Arch Cardiovasc Dis. 2013;106(11):586–92.
33. Gill TM, Allore HG, Han L. Bathing disability and the risk of long-term admission to a nursing home. J Gerontol A Biol Sci Med Sci. 2006;61(8):821–5.
34. Odden MC, Peralta CA, Haan MN, Covinsky KE. Rethinking the association of high blood pressure with mortality in elderly adults: the impact of frailty. Arch Intern Med. 2012;172(15):1162–8.
35. Guralnik JM, Seeman TE, Tinetti ME, Nevitt MC, Berkman LF. Validation and use of performance measures of functioning in a non-disabled older population: MacArthur studies of successful aging. Aging (Milano). 1994;6(6):410–9.
36. Katz S. Assessing self-maintenance: activities of daily living, mobility, and instrumental activities of daily living. J Am Geriatr Soc. 1983;31(12):721–7.

37. Hickson M. Malnutrition and ageing. Postgrad Med J. 2006;82(963):2–8.
38. Mazzola P, Ward L, Zazzetta S, Broggini V, Anzuini A, Valcarcel B, et al. Association between preoperative malnutrition and postoperative delirium after hip fracture surgery in older adults. J Am Geriatr Soc. 2017;65(6):1222–8.
39. Donini LM, Savina C, Rosano A, De Felice MR, Tassi L, De Bernardini L, et al. MNA predictive value in the follow-up of geriatric patients. J Nutr Health Aging. 2003;7(5):282–93.
40. Visvanathan R, Penhall R, Chapman I. Nutritional screening of older people in a sub-acute care facility in Australia and its relation to discharge outcomes. Age Ageing. 2004;33(3):260–5.
41. Bellelli G, Carnevali L, Corsi M, Morandi A, Zambon A, Mazzola P, et al. The impact of psychomotor subtypes and duration of delirium on 6-month mortality in hip-fractured elderly patients. Int J Geriatr Psychiatry. 2018;33:1229.
42. Morandi A, Di Santo SG, Zambon A, Mazzone A, Cherubini A, Mossello E, et al. Delirium, dementia and in-hospital mortality: the results from the Italian Delirium Day 2016, a national multicenter study. J Gerontol A Biol Sci Med Sci. 2018;74:910.
43. Kane RL, Shamliyan T, Talley K, Pacala J. The association between geriatric syndromes and survival. J Am Geriatr Soc. 2012;60(5):896–904.
44. Barr VJ, Robinson S, Marin-Link B, Underhill L, Dotts A, Ravensdale D, et al. The expanded chronic care model: an integration of concepts and strategies from population health promotion and the chronic care model. Hosp Q. 2003;7(1):73–82.
45. Hopman P, Schellevis FG, Rijken M. Health-related needs of people with multiple chronic diseases: differences and underlying factors. Qual Life Res. 2016;25(3):651–60.
46. Chang JH, Vines E, Bertsch H, Fraker DL, Czerniecki BJ, Rosato EF, et al. The impact of a multidisciplinary breast cancer center on recommendations for patient management: the University of Pennsylvania experience. Cancer. 2001;91(7):1231–7.
47. Sainsbury R, Haward B, Rider L, Johnston C, Round C. Influence of clinician workload and patterns of treatment on survival from breast cancer. Lancet. 1995;345(8960):1265–70.
48. Ledwidge M, Barry M, Cahill J, Ryan E, Maurer B, Ryder M, et al. Is multidisciplinary care of heart failure cost-beneficial when combined with optimal medical care? Eur J Heart Fail. 2003;5(3):381–9.
49. Mas M, Inzitari M, Sabaté S, Santaeugènia SJ, Miralles R. Hospital-at-home Integrated Care Programme for the management of disabling health crises in older patients: comparison with bed-based Intermediate Care. Age Ageing. 2017;46(6):925–31.
50. Borrill CS, Carletta J, Carter AJ, Dawson JF, Garrod S, Rees A, Richards A, Shapiro D, West MA. The effectiveness of health care teams in the national health service. Birmingham: University of Aston in Birmingham; 2000. http://homepages.inf.ed.ac.uk/jeanc/DOH-final-report.pdf.
51. Flaherty JE, Hyer K, Fulmer T. Hazzard's geriatric medicine and gerontology. 6th ed. New York: McGraw-Hill Companies; 2009.
52. Royal College of Physicians and Royal College of Nursing. Ward rounds in medicine. 6th ed. London: Royal College of Physicians and Royal College of Nursing; 2012.
53. Leggat SG. Effective healthcare teams require effective team members: defining teamwork competencies. BMC Health Serv Res. 2007;7:17.
54. Mukamel DB, Peterson DR, Temkin-Greener H, Delavan R, Gross D, Kunitz SJ, et al. Program characteristics and enrollees' outcomes in the Program of All-Inclusive Care for the Elderly (PACE). Milbank Q. 2007;85(3):499–531.
55. Coutu D. Why teams don't work. Har Bus Rev. 2009;87:98.
56. Tuckman BW. Developmental sequence in small groups. Psychol Bull. 1965;63(6):384–99. https://psycnet.apa.org/doiLanding?doi=10.1037%2Fh0022100.
57. Taplin SH, Foster MK, Shortell SM. Organizational leadership for building effective health care teams. Ann Fam Med. 2013;11(3):279–81.
58. Mccarthy D, Ryan J, Klein S. Models of care for high-need, high-cost patients: an evidence synthesis. Issue Brief. 2015;31:1.
59. Fossey EM, Harvey CA. A conceptual review of functioning: implications for the development of consumer outcome measures. Aust N Z J Psychiatry. 2001;35(1):91–8.

60. Persson M, Nilsson S, Iwarsson S. Development of multi-disciplinary team I-ADL assessment in community health care: an interrater reliability study of the measure of instrumental daily activity. Arch Gerontol Geriatr. 1999;29(2):149–63.
61. Iwarsson S, Wahl HW, Nygren C, Oswald F, Sixsmith A, Sixsmith J, et al. Importance of the home environment for healthy aging: conceptual and methodological background of the European ENABLE-AGE Project. Gerontologist. 2007;47(1):78–84.
62. Law M, Baptiste S, McColl M, Opzoomer A, Polatajko H, Pollock N. The Canadian occupational performance measure: an outcome measure for occupational therapy. Can J Occup Ther. 1990;57(2):82–7.
63. College of Occupational Therapists Ltd. Reducing the pressure on hospitals: a report on the value of occupational therapy in Scotland. London: College of Occupational Therapists Ltd; 2016. www.COT.co.uk.
64. Townsend E, Polatajko H. Enabling occupation II: advancing an occupational therapy vision for health, well-being & justice through occupation. Ottawa: CAOT Publications ACE; 2007.
65. Parkinson S, Forsyth K, Kielhofner G. Model of human occupation screening tool (MOHOST, version 2.0). University of Illinois: The Model of Human Occupation; 2006.
66. Kielhofner G, Burke JP. A model of human occupation, part 1. Conceptual framework and content. Am J Occup Ther. 1980;34(9):572–81.
67. Kielhofner G. Model of human occupation. 4th ed. Baltimore: Lippincott Williams & Wilkins; 2008.
68. Taylor R. Kielhofner's model of human occupation: theory and application. 5th ed. Philadelphia: Wolters Kluwer; 2017.
69. Fisher A, Jones KB. Assessment of motor and process skills, vol. 1: development, standardization, and administration manual. 7th ed. Fort Collins: Three Star Press; 2012.
70. Fisher A, Jones KB. Assessment of motor and process skills. 8th ed. Fort Collins: Three Star Press; 2014.
71. Fisher A, Atler K, Potts A. Effectiveness of occupational therapy with frail community living older adults. Scand J Occup Ther. 2007;14:240–9.
72. Law M, Baptiste S, Carswell-Opzoomer A, McColl M, Polatajko H, Pollock N. Canadian occupational performance measure manual. 5th ed. Toronto: CAOT Publications ACE; 2014.
73. Enemark Larsen A, Rasmussen B, Christensen JR. Enhancing a client-centred practice with the Canadian occupational performance measure. Occup Ther Int. 2018;2018:5956301.
74. Atwal A, Owen S, Davies R. Struggling for occupational satisfaction: older people in care homes. Br J Occup Ther. 2003;66:118–24.
75. van Seben R, Reichardt L, Smorenburg S, Buurman B. Goal-setting instruments in geriatric rehabilitation: a systematic review. J Frailty Aging. 2017;6(1):37–45.
76. Maritz R, Baptiste S, Darzins SW, Magasi S, Weleschuk C, Prodinger B. Linking occupational therapy models and assessments to the ICF to enable standardized documentation of functioning. Can J Occup Ther. 2018;85:330.
77. Graff MJ, Vernooij-Dassen MJ, Thijssen M, Dekker J, Hoefnagels WH, Rikkert MG. Community based occupational therapy for patients with dementia and their care givers: randomised controlled trial. BMJ. 2006;333(7580):1196.
78. Graff M, Vernooij-Dassen M, Zajec J, Olde Rikkert M, Hoefnagels W, Dekker J. How can occupational therapy improve the daily performance and communication of an older patient with dementia and his primary caregiver? A case study. Dementia. 2006;5:503–32.
79. Pierce D. Occupational science for occupational therapy. Thorofare: Slack Incorporated; 2014.
80. Clark F, Azen SP, Zemke R, Jackson J, Carlson M, Mandel D, et al. Occupational therapy for independent-living older adults. A randomized controlled trial. JAMA. 1997;278(16):1321–6.
81. Clark F, Jackson J, Carlson M, Chou CP, Cherry BJ, Jordan-Marsh M, et al. Effectiveness of a lifestyle intervention in promoting the well-being of independently living older people: results of the Well Elderly 2 Randomised Controlled Trial. J Epidemiol Community Health. 2012;66(9):782–90.
82. Clark F, Blanchard J, Sleight A, Cogan A, Florindez L, Gleason S, editors. Lifestyle Redesign®: the intervention tested in the USC well elderly studies. 2nd ed. Bethesda: AOTA Press; 2015.

Occupational Therapy in the Community

3

Maud J. L. Graff, Lucia Bergamini, Mandy Chamberlain, and Ingrid H. W. M. Sturkenboom

3.1 Introduction

The ageing of populations is rapidly increasing worldwide. However, unfortunately the process of ageing is often associated with chronic disease, such as heart disease, stroke, chronic respiratory disorders, cancer and dementia and a general decline in the intrinsic capacity of the individual [1, 2].

M. J. L. Graff (✉) · I. H. W. M. Sturkenboom
Department Occupational Therapy, Radboud University Medical Center, Nijmegen, The Netherlands

Donders Institute for Brain, Cognition and Behavior, Nijmegen, The Netherlands

Department of Rehabilitation, Scientific Institute for Quality of Healthcare Research, Nijmegen, The Netherlands
e-mail: maud.graff@radboudumc.nl; ingrid.sturkenboom@radboudumc.nl

L. Bergamini
Center for Cognitive Disorders for Adults and Elderly, Mirandola, Italy

Health Local Agency, Modena, Italy

Special Care Unit for Dementia and Behavioural and Psychological Symptoms of Dementia, CISA, Mirandola, Italy
e-mail: l.bergamini@ausl.mo.it

M. Chamberlain
Boulder, CO, USA
e-mail: mchamberlain@seniorsflourish.com

© Springer Nature Switzerland AG 2020
C. Pozzi et al. (eds.), *Occupational Therapy for Older People*,
https://doi.org/10.1007/978-3-030-35731-3_3

There are different trajectories of ageing: normal ageing and accelerated ageing [3]. Healthy ageing is more than just the absence of disease [4]. It can be defined as a process of developing and maintaining the functional ability that enables well-being in older age. This fits with the new definition of health by Huber, in which health is defined as 'the ability to adapt and to self-manage, in the face of social, physical and emotional challenges' [5]. Frailty is highly prevalent in old age and may lead to high risk for falls, disability, hospitalization and mortality. Frailty is not synonymous with either comorbidity or disability, but comorbidity is an etiologic risk factor for frailty, and disability is an outcome of frailty [3].

Moreover, older age frequently involves significant changes beyond biological losses, including shifts in roles and social positions, and the need to deal with the loss of close relationships. In response, older adults tend to select fewer and new meaningful goals and activities, optimize their existing abilities through practice and new technologies and compensate for the losses of some abilities by finding other ways to accomplish tasks. Goals, motivational priorities and preferences may change [6].

Most elderly people find it very important to maintain functional capacity and have a supportive environment. An active life with meaningful activities enables healthy older people, vulnerable older people and older people with disabilities to lead a meaningful life and maintain residual skills.

The general role of the occupational therapist is to support the person and his caregiver to maintain meaningful activities and roles in the domains of self-care, work and leisure activities for as long as possible. When the usual performance is no longer possible, occupational therapists support individuals in adapting the performance method, the activities or the physical and social environment [7]. There are specific skills that characterize the occupational therapists who work in the client's own home environment or in community-based centres. Interpersonal skills are critical for community-based practice and include consulting, staff education/in-services, and advocacy. Equally important is networking, knowledge of community resources, management of volunteers, programme evaluation and multicultural practice issues [8, 9].

Occupational therapy programmes in community are intended for the healthy, frail or disabled elderly. The aim is to maintain or increase the elderly person's residual autonomy, including purposeful and meaningful activities in a social context, rather than focusing on impairments or body structure. The programmes also focus on caregivers, with the aim to reduce stress related to care [10–12]. The attention paid to caregivers and the elderly takes on a significant value since in most European countries, the largest part of elderly people who are not self-sufficient are assisted at home by formal and informal caregivers [13, 14].

Occupational therapy interventions for elderly are occupation-focused with the primary aim to improve occupational performance. Preferably the interventions are also occupation-based, meaning that the clients are engaged in real-life activities and tasks during the assessment and the intervention [10]. In occupation-focused interventions, the acquisitional model and/or the model of adaptive occupation can be used. The outcomes of community-based occupational therapy interventions can be various: falls prevention, maintenance or improvement of ADL and IADL performance, leisure and social participation. Indirectly, occupational therapy may improve health and quality of life and reduce societal costs [15–20].

Although occupational therapy in the community may be involved with individuals or groups with various types of morbidities or disabilities, we will highlight in this chapter some evidence-based programmes for healthy and frail elderly, people with dementia, and people with Parkinson's disease.

Additionally, we will describe the concept and development of dementia friendly community (DFC) to illustrate the importance of the role of the environment in supporting elderly with chronic disease, frail or disabled to feel included in society.

3.2 Community-Based Occupational Therapy in Healthy and Frail Elderly

3.2.1 Background

Occupational therapists can provide services to the well elderly in the community through a shift from a rehabilitative model, where the focus is on services to individuals or groups with a specific limitation or disability, to a broader role. This model promotes areas such as well-being, health promotion and disease prevention to communities and entire populations by implementing group education, which ultimately increases quality of life and the promotion of active ageing.

Programmes that focus on community-based healthy ageing, such as the Ageing Well by Design and Lifestyle Redesign®, look to fill the need through health promotion of community dwelling older adults through community outreach. The programme focuses on occupational engagement, and delays age-related decline in function, increases well-being and ultimately reduces healthcare costs [21, 22].

In comparison to community-based centre programmes, by providing home-based services to frail older adults, occupational therapy practitioners are able to address the client factors, performance skills, and performance patterns that may interfere with the occupations that are necessary for clients to live safely and productively in their home environments after illness, disability or occupational limitation [23]. This helps the individual to stay in their home environment and out of the hospital. This can be achieved through either a short-term intervention, such as a temporary period after a hospitalization, or a long-term intervention, such as an extended period of treatment for people with chronic conditions or increased levels of complexity. This focuses on maintaining a person's highest level of independence, health, assist in chronic disease management, prevent rehospitalisation or hospital-acquired conditions, specifically in the areas of fall prevention and medication management [24].

3.2.2 Healthy Ageing for the Well Elderly Through Prevention

The focus in the Well Elderly Study and the Lifestyle Redesign® programme is on helping older adults recognize the self as an occupational being through redesigning their lifestyle delivered through both individualized and group approaches [25]. It aims to educate on pre-established class material, set personal goals and address sustainable health promoting daily routine for the participants in order to achieve healthy ageing and general well-being.

Lifestyle Redesign® is an activity-based programme that assists participants to implement a personally feasible, healthy lifestyle into their daily lives and daily routines. Intervention includes education on healthy activity, active coping, social support and perceived control of situation. The programme consists of weekly 2 h sessions which are held in a community setting, along with up to ten individual sessions. The programme continues for 9 months if utilizing the Well Elderly I framework or 6 months utilizing the Well Elderly II framework [22].

Each group is led by an occupational therapist and is educated on the intervention modules as illustrated in Table 3.1.

The participants also participate in community education once every 4 weeks for further reinforcement of the provided education, continued exploration and implementation of the new occupations into their daily life.

Although research supports that Lifestyle Redesign® is beneficial and is a cost effective intervention, the majority of healthcare systems in the United States have not adopted this approach due to barriers including funding for preventive services, limited time commitment of participants and shortage of occupational therapy practitioners working in community-based settings [26].

Due to these barriers, most community-based programmes are provided through partnerships between occupational therapists and community organizations. These programmes include multi-component well-being or evidence-based prevention programming completed within a group setting to help older adults maintain their independence, improve occupational performance and promote wellness. Group education can include a variety of topics and education strategies including functional exercises, client education, simulation activities and easily digestible tips to promote health and well-being.

In Table 3.2, examples of community-based group programmes for the well elderly are provided.

Older adults demonstrate an increased risk for decline in physical ability (including ADL participation), mental health and loss of independence. Research supports

Table 3.1 Intervention modules of the lifestyle redesign®

1. Occupation, health and aging
2. Community mobility, transportation and occupation
3. The building blocks of longevity: Various types of activity
4. Stress and inflammation management
5. Dining and nutrition
6. Time and occupation
7. Home and community safety
8. Relationships and occupation
9. Thriving
10. Navigating healthcare
11. Hormones, aging, & sexuality
12. Ending a group—Finalizing personal engagement plans

Table 3.2 Examples of community-based group programmes

• Aging in place programmes
• Caregiver education and support
• CarFit programmes
• Chronic disease management (general education), including
– Arthritis
– Diabetes
– Chronic obstructive pulmonary disease
– Congestive heart failure
– Obesity
• Cognitive programmes to promote brain health
• Community mobility
• Driving and effects of aging on driving abilities
• Energy conservation
• Exercise programmes focusing on strength, balance, and/or flexibility
• Fall prevention
• Home safety/environmental modification
• Leisure programmes specific to cognitive or physical level
• Time management
• Walking programmes

that occupational therapy community-based programmes and education increases the overall health and slows down ageing-related decline for older adults who live in the community better than those that participate in general community social activities [21, 22].

3.2.3 Treatment and Intervention of the Frail Elderly Through Home-Based Occupational Therapy Services

Frailty can be defined as a range of conditions in older people, including general debility and cognitive impairment, that limit occupational performance, increase the prevalence of dependency and have a reduced life expectancy. These deficits may limit their ability to live independently and predispose them to illness and side effects of treatment interventions [27]. The evidence supports that occupational therapy intervention improves functioning of frail older adults living in the community, especially mobility, functioning in daily living activities and social participation, with secondary outcomes included decreased fear of falling, of number of falls, of disability, and improved cognition [18].

3.2.4 Assessment

While working directly in a person's home environment, occupational therapy practitioners are able to complete an interview with the client and/or the client's caregivers to get a good foundation of the client's current occupations, personal interests, occupational history and experiences, patterns of daily living, interests, values and needs. Further the evaluation of the client's home environment and context that supports or barriers to occupational engagement is needed.

Analysis of the client's occupational performance is completed, after looking specifically at the client's strengths, limitations/problems or potential problems. Performance skills, performance patterns, context or environment, client factors and activity demands are all considered, but only selected aspects may be specifically assessed. Because the evaluation is being completed in the individual's own home environment, the occupational therapist is able to directly see how the context and environment affects occupational performance, thus, creating highly individualized client-centred goals.

3.2.5 Treatment

Treatment interventions are specific to the needs of the person who is frail, but the focus is on the individual and caregiver's specific goals and what is meaningful to them in their home environment. Starting with a top-down approach is helpful so that the occupational therapist and client can prioritize and focus on what is most important, relevant or a top occupational priority to address [28].

Case Study
Ms. Miller is a 76-year-old woman receiving home health occupational therapy services after experiencing a fall in the shower, resulting in a total hip arthroplasty. She has poorly controlled diabetes, which has resulted in peripheral neuropathy of her feet. She reports that since returning home, her pain has been up to a seven out of ten, and because of this, she has been staying in bed since returning home.

She enjoys going to the local senior centre each week to play cards with her friends. She reports enjoying completing the household chores such as laundry and cooking meals.

She lives in a one-story home with her husband, who is able to assist in her care, but is struggling physically to get around the home himself. Ms. Miller is alert and oriented, but her husband reports that she has some forgetfulness and she sometimes forgets to take her medications.

The occupational therapist and the client decide that preventing further falls, controlling pain and getting in the shower are the client's top priorities. They start with adaptive equipment recommendations such as a grab bar, non-skid tape on the floor and shower chair in the shower, as well as educating her in safe use of the walker into the bathroom for shower transfers.

They also began working on medication management by establishing a routine with alarms set throughout the day so she will remember to take her pain medications as prescribed and began diabetes management education.

There will be an increased need for community-based occupational therapy services as the older adult population grows, individuals age in place, maintain their independence and participate in an active lifestyle. Occupational therapy will be a crucial link in the success of this population achieving these goals as it offers the solution to occupational participation, health promotion and well-being for healthy and frail older adults in the community.

3.3 The Community Occupational Therapy in Dementia Programme (COTiD-Programme)

3.3.1 Background

The *Community Occupational Therapy in Dementia programme (COTiD-programme)* for clients with dementia and their caregivers is a multi-component, individualized and tailored client-and-caregiver-centred (system-centred) intervention programme. The COTiD-programme enables clients with dementia to participate in meaningful daily activities in their own environment and enables caregivers to effectively support them in these activities. It is also focused on the participation in meaningful activities and reducing the burden of their caregivers [29]. The overall aim is to improve the quality of life and health of both the clients with dementia and their caregivers.

The effectiveness of community-based occupational therapy for older people with dementia and their caregivers was evaluated in a randomized controlled trial in the Netherlands [13, 20]. The intervention was proven effective in improving the participants' daily functioning (improved skills (AMPS) and decreased need for assistance (IDDD)), health, mood and quality of life, and the caregiver's sense of competence (SCQ). The results were supported by the same effective intervention components of Gitlin et al. [30] and Leven et al. [31].

Moreover, community-based occupational therapy was found to be cost-effective in terms of a significant high proportion of successful treatments and a decrease of costs of health care consumption from a societal perspective [15]. Successful treatment was based on a clinically relevant improvement on all three primary outcomes measures: on clients' skills in daily functioning, on client's need for assistance and on the feeling of competence in the caregivers. The ten intervention sessions based on the COTiD-programme saved 1750 euro per client and caregiver couple that was treated successfully [15].

3.3.2 Content of the COTiD Programme

The COTiD programme is focused on conducting optimal adaptation of the limitations related to the presence of dementia. The aims are to train and coach the problem-solving, coping and supervision skills of the caregivers and the effective use of strategies by the people with dementia (PWD) in meaningful everyday activities. In this person-caregiver-centred intervention, the caregiver acts as the expert of his own caregiving situation. The occupational therapist has different roles: (1) the role of a trainer/teacher and (2) the role of a coach. The intervention goals are focused on improving the performance and participation in meaningful daily activities of both people and the coping, problem-solving and supervision skills of the caregiver. This intervention approach is based on the model of human occupation (MOHO) [32], narrative interviewing methods [33], the Ethnographic Framework of Gitlin [34], and the problem-solving process and self-management model of Lorig [35].

The information from the PWDs and caregivers stories, their beliefs, needs, interests, habits, roles, norms and goals, their self-perceived efficacy, the observations of the occupational therapist of their use of skills and strategies in familiar daily activities and the possibilities of the physical and social environment, are summarized for use in the shared goal-setting and intervention processes. During the intervention the occupational therapist trains the PWD to make effective use of their remaining skills and strategies and coaches caregivers to solve problems by following the phases of the problem-solving circle, which is based on the self-management model of Lorig et al. [35], including how to adapt the physical and social environment to the consequences of dementia in daily life. They are also coached to focus on their own participation in meaningful activities. The COTiD-programme consists of ten intervention sessions (once or twice a week) which are conducted at the PWD's home [29, 36]. The intervention is directed at all people with mild to moderate dementia, who are living in the community, and at their informal caregivers (partners, family members, neighbours or friends) who support them at least 1 day a week. The intervention can also be delivered at people living in homes for the elderly and their professional and informal caregivers.

The COTiD-programme contains of three intervention phases as illustrated in Table 3.3.

Case Study
Mr. Smith is 71 years old and lives with his wife in a self-built bungalow. Last week he was told that he has mild dementia. Besides this, he has decreased mobility due to his hip problems. He hopes that he and his wife can live independently for as long as possible in their own bungalow. Mr. Smith says that he does not experience problems at the moment. However, he reports that he has problems with starting up activities, he is getting a bit slower than he used to be and he says that he recently had some problems with driving a car and cooking a meal. His 70 years old wife takes care of the husband and she is complaining of back pain due to the care overload. However, in some ways, she feels better since her husband has been diagnosed with dementia because she can better understand his behaviour but she is afraid of the future and the consequences related to the presence of dementia.

The occupational therapist uses the life story assessments (OPHI and Ethnographic Interview) in her talk to Mr. and Mrs. Smith separately, and observes meaningful activities that Mr. Smith is used to perform with or without assistance of Mrs. Smith. In the next meeting the occupational therapist discusses the wishes of Mr. and Mrs. Smith for performing meaningful activities from the two stories, and

Table 3.3 Content and process of the COTiD-programme

Phase A: The strength, needs and case formulation phase (four 1-h-sessions)	Story of the older person with dementia	Daily routines inventory OPHI narrative interview: Insight in person with dementia' interests, believes, habits, roles, important activities, self-efficacy, physical, social environment; of the past, present and future
	Story of the informal caregiver (CG)	Daily routines inventory Ethnographic narrative interview: Insight in CG' interests, believes, habits, roles, important activities, self-efficacy, physical, social environment; of the past, present and future and insight in caregiving role, use of coping strategies, and care capacity, needs for support
	Story of the occupational therapist	Physical environment inventory Observation of daily activities by the Assessment of Motor & Process Skills (AMPS) Observation of Communication & Interactions Skills by Assessment of Communication and Interaction Skills (ACIS) Summary & Interpretation of the three stories of Phase A on Form
Phase B: Goal setting phase (one 1-h session)	Summary of the three stories	Wishes and meaningful activities of person with dementia, of CG, and interpretation of stories and observations by occupational therapist
	Choosing and prioritizing most meaningful goals on goals setting form and scoring COPM performance & satisfaction	Goals for person with dementia Goals for CG Goals for both people together COPM scoring person with dementia COPM scoring CG
Phase C: Implementation of the intervention plan and evaluation phase (five 1-h-sessions)	Treatment phase of person with dementia, CG and both people together	Observing strategies person with dementia Problem-solving CG: Self-management coaching Plan, perform and evaluate interventions on different goals person with dementia & CG on goals & COPM form

the conclusions from the observations and educates about the dementia and its consequences for daily life related to the activities mentioned. She asks them separately and together to prioritize their most important meaningful activities. The occupational therapist together with Mr. and Mrs. Smith formulates goals for improving these prioritized meaningful activities. Accordingly, the occupational therapist asks them to score these goals in terms of their current performance, and their satisfaction with this performance. The aims of the COTiD treatment accordingly are: (a) Improving Mr. Smith's skills through adaptation of the environment (like memory aids, instructions, simplifying the environment) and using his most effective strategies in an efficient way to perform his prioritized meaningful activities; (b) Improving Mrs Smith's problem-solving and coping skills. According to the problem-solving model, six steps are followed. (1) Mrs. Smith and the occupational therapist agree that Mrs. Smith is the expert of her own caregiving situation. She is together with the occupational therapist responsible to find suitable solutions for the problems they are faced to. (2) Together with Mrs Smith the occupational therapist observes and analyses Mr. Smith when performing his prioritized meaningful daily activities (preparing the vegetables and gardening)—what strategies he uses and which are effective. (3) Following this, the occupational therapist meets with Mrs Smith alone and coaches Mrs Smith to describe and analyse what the problem in one of the activities is. (4) And to discuss what they have tried already, evaluate how it worked out. (5) Accordingly Mrs. Smith is asked to look for feasible alternatives to perform this activity in an effective way. (6) After this, she is coached by the occupational therapist to find a possible solution, the occupational therapist therefore uses the sentence 'How Could You Achieve that…'. Solutions can be effective ways of adapting or preparing the task, simplifying the environment, using effective cues and ways of approaching Mr. Smith. (7) Accordingly they decide Mrs. Smith will perform the activities accordingly to this possible solution together with Mr. Smith during the week. (8) Afterwards the occupational therapist and Mrs. Smith meet again and evaluate how this possible solution worked out. If it did not work out well they start the problem-solving model again, and probably carry out the activity with Mr. Smith Mrs. Smith and the occupational therapist together, until a feasible solution is found. Accordingly, they go through the problem-solving model and look for solutions for the goal of Mrs. Smith: 'to find more time to perform her own meaningful activities'. At the end of the treatment period, the occupational therapist evaluates with both people the treatment goals on the goal-setting form again. They discuss the results achieved and end the occupational therapy.

3.3.3   National and Cross-National Implementation

At this moment, COTiD is translated in four different languages (German research version, Voigt-Radloff), French [37], English [38], Italian [39]. The COTiD is being implemented in all these countries by training teachers according to a train-the-trainer-programme and supervision of the implementation on a consult basis in all six countries. These are respectively Germany, France, the UK, Italy, Switzerland and the Netherlands. The COTiD-programme was proven (cost-) effective in a randomized controlled trial in the Netherlands [13, 15, 20]. However, this was not found in a German pragmatic multicentre trial [40, 41]. Explanations for these results were that COTiD was not adapted to the German culture before this intervention was implemented and evaluated for effectiveness. Moreover, occupational therapists had no experience and limited training in the programme before start of the pragmatic randomized controlled trial in German routine care. Cultural differences in client–caregiver and professional characteristics as also implementation problems played an important role [40, 41]. In the Netherlands, by implementing COTiD in routine care nationwide strategies were used, but they appeared to be partly effective. This was due to barriers in bridging the gap between research and practice, like quality of professional networks, professional and organizational barriers [42–44]. This was also found in other implementation studies of effective programmes in routine care. At the moment, COTiD is implemented well in the Netherlands, about 70% of occupational therapists working with persons with dementia at home are trained in the COTiD and collaborate in regional groups. The new COTiD training has added coaching on the job additionally and ways to deal with difficult situation and how to implement COTiD best in these regional group are discussed during the course and the regional groups. It was found that cross-national implementation needs a careful preparative process. It is important to first translate the programme and accordingly develop country specific COTiD-programme adaptation, second to get understanding on access to and quality of care delivery and third on barriers and facilitators for effective implementation, implementation strategies and intervening factors before effectively implementing evidence-based psychosocial interventions, like COTiD, in other countries [45]. In the UK a research project is being carried out where they try to follow these steps for cross-national implementation [46]. In a pilot study in Italy, positive changes were found. Both the person with dementia's and caregivers' self-perceived performance and satisfaction in daily activities and caregivers' sense of competence showed significant positive changes after COTiD delivered in an uncontrolled study to clients with mild to moderate dementia and caregivers [14].

3.4   Community Occupational Therapy in Parkinson's Disease

3.4.1   Background

Parkinson's disease is a neurodegenerative disorder that progressively affects the dopaminergic and non-dopaminergic areas of the brain [47]. Parkinson's disease is the fastest growing neurodegenerative disorder and the number of persons with PD worldwide is expected to double, from 6.9 to 14.2 million by 2040 [48]. It is not necessarily a disease of old age, but prevalence rises with increasing age.

The disease leads to a complex and individual pattern of motor- and non-motor symptoms. Cardinal motor symptoms are bradykinesia, rigidity and tremor. Postural instability is a cardinal feature in more advanced disease stages. Examples of possible non-motor symptoms are depression, cognitive impairments, anxiety and sleep disorders. The disease progressively impacts on the ability of persons with Parkinson's disease to engage in meaningful daily activities. An individually tailored and multifaceted approach to care is warranted. The focus of occupational therapists is to support persons with Parkinson's disease and their caregivers to face challenges in engaging in meaningful activities and roles.

Evidence for the effectiveness of community-based occupational therapy interventions in Parkinson's disease is scarce. In this section we will summarize the evidence and contents for an individualized community-based occupational therapy intervention for persons with Parkinson's disease and their caregivers, called *the*

OTiP-intervention. The OTiP-intervention has been developed and researched in the Netherlands and is based on the Dutch clinical guideline for occupational therapy in Parkinson's disease [49, 50]. The impact and effectiveness of the OTiP-intervention was systematically assessed in consecutively a feasibility study and a full scale randomized controlled trial. The trial demonstrated that the OTiP-intervention was effective in improving self-perceived performance in prioritized occupational performance issues [51]. In the economic evaluation, no significant differences in total costs were found over a 6 months period, but there were significant savings on institutional care in the intervention group [17]. The process evaluation showed that the individual tailoring of the intervention to the needs, wishes and capabilities of the patient and possibilities of the context is a particular strength of the intervention. Though, the therapists experienced this tailoring as challenging [52].

3.4.2   Content of the OTiP-Intervention

The OTiP-intervention is client-centred, occupation-focused and addresses the needs of both the person with Parkinson's disease and the caregiver. Knowledge about the disease is needed to take into account Parkinson-specific problems in the assessment and treatment.

In Table 3.4 an overview is given of the process and elements of the OTiP-intervention.

3.4.2.1 The Assessment Phase

Important in this phase are the narrative interview style to identify values, strengths, needs and priorities in relation to occupational performance. Themes from the Occupational Performance History Interview (OPHI-II) [33] are used, as well as the Canadian Occupational Performance Interview (COPM) [53]. A separate narrative interview is conducted with the partner or main informal caregiver, to recognize their strengths, needs and own well-being in supporting and supervising the person with Parkinson's disease in daily activities. Additionally, the person is observed while performing a goal-directed meaningful activity in the context that is sufficiently challenging from a motor and cognitive point of view. Therapists preferably use a generic validated and standardized assessment for observation, like the Assessment of Motor and Process Skills (AMPS) [54] or the Perceive Recall Plan Perform system of Task Analysis (PRPP assessment) [55]. If the client experiences medication related response fluctuations, the occupational therapist should be aware to get a good evaluation of occupational performance and specific issues in the *on* and the *off* phase.

3.4.2.2 Collaborative Goal Setting and Treatment Planning

The goals and potential intervention strategies are individually tailored guided by findings from the assessment phase. In early stages of Parkinson's disease, goals mainly include restoring or maintaining 'normal' occupational performance. In

Table 3.4 The process and elements of the OTiP-intervention

Assessment (2–3 sessions)
1. Establish occupational profile (values, needs) and context (narrative interview)
2. Identify/prioritize main occupational issues for both person with Parkinson's disease *and* caregiver
3. Explore context and coping related to prioritized issues
4. Observe quality of occupational performance and performance skills in natural environment
5. Evaluate environmental factors
6. Collect information on underlying impairments as appropriate
Collaborative goal setting and treatment planning
Treatment
Variety of strategies or advices tailored to individual needs
Possible interventions for person with Parkinson's disease
• Stimulating self-management, education/coaching
• Training 'normal 'performance skills (restore, maintain)
• Compensatory strategies to improve task performance such as
– Parkinson-specific movement strategies: Focused attention, sensory cues and reorganizing complex performance sequences
– Cognitive rehabilitation strategies
– Energy management strategies
• Advice on optimizing daily routines and simplifying activities
• Advice on appropriate aids and adaptations
Possible interventions for caregiver
• Provision of information (impact of disease on daily functioning of patient, possible care resources, aids and adaptations)
• Training supervision skills
Evaluation of achievement of goals and/or need to adjust plan

later stages of disease this will shift towards enabling adapted involvement in valued activities. Often a combination of intervention strategies is used to work on specific goals. The interventions can be directed at the person, the activity or the environment. In the guideline the Person-Environment-Occupation model [56] is used to categorize the interventions.

3.4.2.3 Treatment Phase

In this phase the treatment plan is implemented. The possible intervention strategies are listed in Table 3.4. Specific to Parkinson's disease are compensatory strategies that facilitate fluency and amplitude of movement, such as focused attention (internal cue) and external sensory cueing. The proposed working mechanism for these strategies is that the impaired neural circuit of movement regulation involving the basal ganglia is bypassed by using other, intact brain areas [57]. Examples of cues are a visual stripe to step over when walking through the door, counting to regulate initiation of a large movement (e.g. when pulling up trousers), marching to keep fluency when turning. Other compensatory strategies that can be used to improve occupational performance in people with Parkinson's disease are strategies derived from the fields of fatigue management and cognitive rehabilitation.

As part of compensation for limitations in activities, the complexity or the timing aspects of the activity itself can be adapted to make the activity less demanding for the person.

Especially in Parkinson's disease, environmental factors impact on functional movement in activities. For example, a confined space provokes freezing. Some environmental adaptations may be required early on in disease, but the need for environmental adaptations will increase as the disease progresses.

For people with Parkinson's disease, the capacity for generalization of learned strategies is more difficult and therefore it is important to focus on functionally important tasks and the familiar performance context. Apart from education and coaching, intervention strategies for the caregiver may extend to actual training of specific handling or supervision skills needed to support the patient.

Case Study

Mr. B lives alone in an apartment. He has had Parkinson's disease for 8 years and is in the moderate disease stage. Mr. B liked to play billiard with his friends in a club near his home. His daughter usually takes him there. Lately he is not so keen to go anymore. The assessment reveals he has freezing of gait when needing to initiate steps around the pool table, he does not strike the ball hard enough due to difficulty with timing the movement. He feels self-conscious towards his friends. Moreover, he often feels fatigued and then cannot be bothered to go. The occupational therapists discusses with him the planning of the activity in the week and how to ensure he has some rest before going to the club to play. In collaboration with the physiotherapist, the occupational therapist explores with Mr. B what are the best external cueing strategies to enhance the stepping and striking movements. A rocking movement before taking a step with focussed attention was most effective. For the striking it helped him to count from 1 to 3 before hitting the ball. The occupational therapist practised the strategies with Mr. B at the club. Mr. B informed his friends of the strategies and the fact that he needs some more time and attention when it is his turn.

3.4.3   Implementation

In the Netherlands, persons with Parkinson's are usually seen by occupational therapists affiliated to ParkinsonNet, a series of regional networks of health professionals specialized in PD [58]. ParkinsonNet offers a unique opportunity for implementing the guideline and the latest evidence on occupational therapy in Parkinson's disease through training, interactive meetings and online sharing of information. The originally Dutch guideline has been translated in English [50] and Italian [59]. The ParkinsonNet concept and basic training is currently also being implemented in parts of the USA, Norway and Luxembourg. The complete implementation in all these countries involved a feasibility study to gain insight in what is needed to tailor the ParkinsonNet concept to the relevant local context, advise a local project team, conduct an initial training course for therapists and offer a train the trainer curriculum.

3.5 Dementia Friendly Communities

3.5.1 Background

The concept of dementia friendliness is beguilingly simple, namely, to work for the common goal of a better life for people with dementia and their families, so they feel included and can participate in society. But it is much more than this. The framework of dementia friendliness has the power to change the way we think about living well with dementia.

Due to cognitive disabilities and social stigma with dementia, people with dementia often refrain from social participation. They show (increasingly) impairments in social skills, taking initiative, behaviour and functioning, even at the very early stages of the disease [60, 61]. People with dementia encounter difficulties in activities of daily living, social relation with others and community activities and hence become socially isolated [62, 63].

Besides stigma, an important explanation for restrictions in social participation is that services do not accommodate to impairments related to dementia and that organizations lack collaboration in meeting the needs of people with dementia. Persons with dementia become confused when trying to be active in a non-dementia friendly society with services that do not accommodate their abilities in non-supportive physical environments like supermarkets, banks, sporting facilities or public transport [64]. Dementia interferes with the positive health of persons with dementia and their informal caregivers. Being a family caregiver for someone with cognitive problems causes burden and stress, and may also result in social isolation underlining the need for carers' support as well [65, 66]. For instance, carers are relieved when those they care for participate in outdoor activities, as this allows them the opportunity to participate in activities on their own [67]. Empowering self-management and inclusion of persons with dementia and carers in meaningful activities appear to be partly effective in enhancing their social participation [64, 68]. Health and welfare interventions, however, are merely offered for a limited time and are not part of daily life. This is why the concept of dementia friendly communities (DFC) has evolved.

The objective of dementia friendly communities is to reduce stigma, increase understanding of dementia by spreading awareness and meaningful engagement for persons with dementia of all ages, empower persons with dementia by recognizing their rights and capabilities so that they feel respected and empower them to take decisions about their life. DFC is a community where persons with dementia can participate in society as long as possible, where the local government makes tailor-made support possible for people with dementia and their caregivers, and increases the knowledge of dementia in their own local government and the whole community, like the offering of a training 'how to deal with dementia' for their employees and citizens. In this way an inclusive community is created in which everybody accepts dementia, from the bakery to the neighbour or the sports club and police agent. Where people with dementia can do shopping, financial activities, go to a club, library or museum. And where the community will assist them where needed.

Engaging people with dementia in the dementia friendly projects, and providing dementia friendly communities means people with dementia can be empowered to live their pre-diagnosis lives for as long as possible, and support them not to give up despite the diagnosis [69].

In recent years, many countries have invested and developed programmes to create communities and friendly activities for dementia, aimed at reducing stigma and supporting people with dementia. This was possible thanks to the involvement of family associations, including people with dementia, institutions and partnerships.

At this moment there is no evaluation review or effect study on the success of DFC in the Netherlands or internationally. Therefore, in 2018 a research started at the Radboud University medical center of Nijmegen in collaboration with the South University for Applied Science and the University of Nottingham to the underlyingh factors and mechanisms of succesful dementia friendly societies. Results of this project are not available yet. We will illustrate in the paragraphs below the experiences of dementia friendly communities in Italy, the Netherlands and the USA so far.

3.5.2   Dementia Friendly Communities in Italy

In Italy in 2016, the biggest national non-profit organization for people with dementia (Federazione Alzheimer Italia), in collaboration with Alzheimer's UK Society, started a pilot study for the first 'Dementia-Friendly Community' project. The choice was driven both by the number of inhabitants and by the fact that this city was already a friendly city with a great culture of solidarity, as demonstrated by the large number of voluntary associations and initiatives. First of all an analysis of the needs of the community was made by a multidisciplinary working group with the aim to evaluate how people living with dementia and their carers perceive the degree of inclusiveness. Focus groups with a selected group of people living with dementia and their carers evaluated efficacy and appropriateness of the different items. At the same time some initiatives like informative events for the whole population, training courses for local police or small traders and civil servants are scheduled [70]. Since 2016 several Italian cities have begun the process of becoming dementia friendly.

3.5.3   Dementia Friendly Communities in the Netherlands

Together Dementia Friendly (*in Dutch* 'Samen dementievriendelijk') is a collaboration of the Dutch Alzheimer Association (Alzheimer Nederland), the Dutch Pension Organisation (PGGM) and the Ministry of Health and Sport, which is part of the Dutch Plan on Dementia (*in Dutch* the Deltaplan Dementie). Their slogan is: 'How we as a community deal with dementia is an important issue. People with dementia are the first years in their disease process very well able to maintain their self-reliance. It is important for them to participate in society as long as possible.'

On their website they provide training materials and interesting educational brochures.

There are many DFC initiatives running in different cities and villages, in all regions of the Netherlands. These are DFC initiatives, like DF tennis club and other sports clubs, hotels, restaurants, shops, all generation public gardens, dental care facilities, choirs, training of: care workers, local government employees, employees of companies, shop workers, bus drivers and also all citizens.

3.5.4   Dementia Friendly Communities in the United States

The organization 'Dementia Friendly America®' was established after the White House Conference on Aging created a call to action to increase dementia friendly initiatives across the United States (US). This was after Minnesota's successful initiative, ACT on Alzheimer's, was developed, creating 34 communities in their home state as 'dementia friendly' [71]. More than 50 organizations across the US have joined this initiative and are working to make dementia friendly communities a reality [72].

Through this national organization, cities from across the US are able to take Dementia Friendly America's community toolkit and duplicate it. This creates a consistent framework.

3.5.5   The Role of Occupational Therapy in DFC

Currently, research does not support occupational therapy in dementia friendly community initiatives, but it is thought that occupational therapy could play an integral role in DFC through:

- Helping people with dementia and family associations to become aware of their needs through the use of structured interviews and focus groups.
- Training members of the community to adopt best practices towards people with dementia.
- Evaluating the environment and providing suggestions and proposals for adaptation.
- Promoting occupation-based programmes for people with dementia aimed at preventing or coping with disability.
- Supporting and educating caregivers to better care for people with dementia.
- Assisting people with dementia in community integration, such as independence in community mobility and adaptive driving.

In the context of DFC it is logical to think that the expertise and competencies of occupational therapists can be a cornerstone in the projects to enable meaningful participation of people with dementia and their caregivers. Working with people, with the community, with organizations is one of the tasks of the occupational therapist. In the future, it is therefore desirable that the role of the occupational therapist can be better exploited in these community enabling contexts. New scientific studies could explore the added value of the role of occupational therapists in a DFC.

Key Messages

- Occupational therapy for elderly in the community maintain residual abilities during the aging process.
- Occupational therapy for elderly in the community is necessary to assist in keeping people independent and in their own homes for as long as possible.
- Occupational therapy for elderly in the community may include services for individuals (including caregivers) and groups.
- Occupational therapy for elderly in the community can focus on prevention, rehabilitation and enablement.
- An occupation-based and client-centred approach is essential to suit the needs of elderly in the community.

References

1. Steves CJ, Spector TD, Jackson SH. Ageing, genes, environment and epigenetics: what twin studies tell us now, and in the future. Age Ageing. 2012;41(5):581–6.
2. Vasto S, Scapagnini G, Bulati M, Candore G, Castiglia L, Colonna-Romano G, et al. Biomarkers of aging. Front Biosci (Schol Ed). 2010;2:392–402.
3. Fried LP, Tangen CM, Walston J, Newman AB, Hirsch C, Gottdiener J, et al. Frailty in older adults: evidence for a phenotype. J Gerontol A Biol Sci Med Sci. 2001;56(3):M146–56.
4. Beard JR, Officer AM, Cassels AK. The world report on ageing and health. Gerontologist. 2016;56(Suppl 2):S163–6.
5. Huber M, Knottnerus JA, Green L, van der Horst H, Jadad AR, Kromhout D, et al. How should we define health? BMJ. 2011;343:d4163.
6. Carstensen LL. The influence of a sense of time on human development. Science. 2006;312(5782):1913–5.
7. Dixon L, Duncan D, Johnson P, Kirkby L, O'Connell H, Taylor H, et al. Occupational therapy for patients with Parkinson's disease. Cochrane Database Syst Rev. 2007;3:CD002813. https://doi.org/10.1002/14651858.CD002813.pub2.
8. Lemorie L, Paul S. Professional expertise of community-based occupational therapists. Occup Ther Health Care. 2001;13(3-4):33–50.
9. Winstead SR. What's in the fridge? Unique competencies of community-based occupational therapists. Open J Occup Ther. 2016;4(4):Article 12.
10. Fisher AG. Occupation-centred, occupation-based, occupation-focused: same, same or different? Scand J Occup Ther. 2013;20(3):162–73.
11. Polatajko HJ, Davis JA. Advancing occupation-based practice: interpreting the rhetoric. Can J Occup Ther. 2012;79(5):259–62.
12. Nagayama H, Tomori K, Ohno K, Takahashi K, Ogahara K, Sawada T, et al. Effectiveness and cost-effectiveness of occupation-based occupational therapy using the aid for decision making in occupation choice (ADOC) for older residents: pilot cluster randomized controlled trial. PLoS One. 2016;11(3):e0150374.
13. Graff MJL, Vernooij-Dassen MJFJ, Thijssen M, OldeRikkert, MGM, Hoefnagels WHL, Dekker J. Community occupational therapy for dementia patients and their primary caregivers: a randomized controlled trial. BMJ. 2006; 333(7580):1196. https://doi.org/10.1136/bmj.39001.688843.BE.
14. Pozzi C, Lanzoni A, Lucchi E, Bergamini L, Bevilacqua P, Manni B, et al. A pilot study of community-based occupational therapy for persons with dementia (COTID-IT Program) and their caregivers: evidence for applicability in Italy. Aging Clin Exp Res. 2018;31(9):1299–304.

15. Graff MJL, Adang EMM, Vernooij-Dassen MJM, Dekker J, Jönsson L, Thijssen M, Hoefnagels WHL, OldeRikkert MGM. Community occupational therapy for older patients with dementia and their caregivers: a cost-effectiveness study. BMJ, 2008;336(7636):134–8. https://doi.org/10.1136/bmj.39408.481898.BE.
16. Gitlin LN, Harris LF, McCoy MC, Chernett NL, Pizzi LT, Jutkowitz E, et al. A home-based intervention to reduce depressive symptoms and improve quality of life in older African Americans: a randomized trial. Ann Intern Med. 2013;159(4):243–52.
17. Sturkenboom IH, Hendriks JC, Graff MJ, Adang EM, Munneke M, Nijhuis-van der Sanden MW, et al. Economic evaluation of occupational therapy in Parkinson's disease: a randomized controlled trial. Mov Disord. 2015;30(8):1059–67.
18. De Coninck L, Bekkering GE, Bouckaert L, Declercq A, Graff MJL, Aertgeerts B. Home- and community-based occupational therapy improves functioning in frail older people: a systematic review. J Am Ger Soc. 2017;65(8):1863–9.
19. Nielsen TL, Petersen KS, Nielsen CV, Strom J, Ehlers MM, Bjerrum M. What are the short-term and long-term effects of occupation-focused and occupation-based occupational therapy in the home on older adults' occupational performance? A systematic review. Scand J Occup Ther. 2017;24(4):235–48.
20. Graff MJ, Vernooij-Dassen MJ, Thijssen M, Dekker J, Hoefnagels WH, Olderikkert MG. Effects of community occupational therapy on quality of life, mood, and health status in dementia patients and their caregivers: a randomized controlled trial. J Gerontol A Biol Sci Med Sci. 2007;62(9):1002–9.
21. Clark F, Azen SP, Zemke R, Jackson J, Carlson M, Mandel D, et al. Occupational therapy for independent-living older adults. A randomized controlled trial. JAMA. 1997;278(16):1321–6.
22. Clark F, Jackson J, Carlson M, Chou CP, Cherry BJ, Jordan-Marsh M, et al. Effectiveness of a lifestyle intervention in promoting the well-being of independently living older people: results of the well elderly 2 randomised controlled trial. J Epidemiol Community Health. 2012;66(9):782–90.
23. American Occupational Therapy Association. Occupational therapy practice framework: domain and process (3rd edition). Am J Occup Ther. 2017;68(Suppl 1):S1–S48.
24. Roberts PS, Robinson MR. Occupational therapy's role in preventing acute readmissions. Am J Occup Ther. 2014;68(3):254–9.
25. Cassidy TB, Richards LG, Eakman AM. Feasibility of a lifestyle redesign®-inspired intervention for well older adults. Am J Occup Ther. 2017;71(4):7104190050p1–6.
26. Clark F, Park DJ, Burke JP. Dissemination: bringing translational research to completion. Am J Occup Ther. 2013;67(2):185–93.
27. Lally F, Crome P. Understanding frailty. Postgrad Med J. 2007;83(975):16–20.
28. Radomski MV, Trombley CA. Occupational therapy for physical dysfunction by Radomski. Philadelphia: Lippincott Williams and Wilkins; 2013.
29. Graff MJL, Vernooij-Dassen MJM, Zajec J, Olde-Rikkert MGM, Hoefnagels WHL, Dekker J. How can occupational therapy improve the daily performance and communication of an older patient with dementia and his primary caregiver? Dementia. 2006;5(4):503–32.
30. Gitlin LN, Hauck WW, Dennis MP, Winter L. Maintenance of effects of the home environmental skill-building program for family caregivers and individuals with Alzheimer's disease and related disorders. J Gerontol A Biol Sci Med Sci. 2005;60(3):368–74.
31. Van't Leven N, Prick AE, Groenewoud JG, Roelofs PD, de Lange J, Pot AM. Dyadic interventions for community-dwelling people with dementia and their family caregivers: a systematic review. Int Psychogeriatr. 2013;25(10):1581–603.
32. Kielhofner G. Model of human occupation. Theory and application. Philadelphia: Lippincott Williams & Wilkins; 2002.
33. Kielhofner G, Mallinson T, Crawford C, Nowak M, Rigby M, Henry A, et al. A User's manual for the occupational performance history interview (version 2.0), OPHI-II. Chicago: The Model of Human Occupation Clearinghouse, Department of Occupational Therapy, College of Applied Health Sciences, UIC: University of Illinois; 2004.

34. Gitlin LN, Corcoran M, Leinmiller-Echhart S. Understanding the family perspective: an ethnographic framework for providing occupational therapy in the home. Am J Occup Ther. 1995;49(8):802–9.
35. Lorig K, Sobel D, Ritter P, Laurent D, Hobbs M. Effect of a self-management program on patients with chronic disease. Eff Clin Pract. 2001;4:256–62.
36. Graff M, Melick M, Thijssen M, Zajec J. Ergotherapie bij ouderen met dementie en hun mantelozrgers: het EDOMAH-programma [Community occupational therapy for older people with dementia and their caregivers. The COTiD program]. Houten: Bohn Stafleu van Loghum; 2010.
37. Graff M, van Melick M, Thijssen M, Verstraten P, Zajec J. L'ergothérapie à domicile auprès des personnes âgées souffrant de démence et leurs aidants [Community occupational therapy for older people with dementia and their caregivers. COTiD programme]. Belgian: Edition DeBoek; 2013. [n French] ISBN: 978-2-35327-188-7.
38. Wenborn J, Graff MJL, Orrell M. Community occupational therapy in Dementia UK (COTiD-UK). Translated and adapted COTiD Manual draft research version. 2013.
39. Graff MJL. Melick M van, Thijssen M, Verstraten P, Zajec J. Curare la demenza a domicilio. Indicazioni di terapia occupazionale per anziani e caregivers. Milano: Franco Angeli; 2016. ISBN 978-88-917-272-2. COTiD-It. [In Italian]. [Italian translation of Community occupational therapy for older people with dementia and their caregivers: COTiD-It].
40. Voigt-Radloff S, Graff M, Leonhart R, Schornstein K, Jessen F, Bohlken J, et al. A multicentre RCT on community occupational therapy in Alzheimer's disease: 10 sessions are not better than one consultation. BMJ Open. 2011;1(1):e000096.
41. Voigt-Radloff S, Graff M, Leonhart R, Hull M, Rikkert MO, Vernooij-Dassen M. Why did an effective Dutch complex psycho-social intervention for people with dementia not work in the German healthcare context? Lessons learnt from a process evaluation alongside a multicentre RCT. BMJ Open. 2011;1(1):e000094.
42. Döpp CM, Graff MJ, Teerenstra S, Adang E, Nijhuis-van der Sanden RW, Olderikkert MG, et al. A new combined strategy to implement a community occupational therapy intervention: designing a cluster randomized controlled trial. BMC Geriatr. 2011;11:13.
43. Dopp CM, Graff MJ, Rikkert MG, Nijhuis van der Sanden MW, Vernooij-Dassen MJ. Determinants for the effectiveness of implementing an occupational therapy intervention in routine dementia care. Implement Sci. 2013;8:131.
44. Dopp CM, Graff MJ, Teerenstra S, Nijhuis-van der Sanden MW, Olde Rikkert MG, Vernooij-Dassen MJ. Effectiveness of a multifaceted implementation strategy on physicians' referral behavior to an evidence-based psychosocial intervention in dementia: a cluster randomized controlled trial. BMC Fam Pract. 2013;14:70.
45. Graff MJL. Community occupational therapy in older people with dementia and their caregivers in the Netherlands and Europe. Jpn Occup Ther Research J. 2015;34:2.
46. Wenborn J, Hynes S, Moniz-Cook E, Mountain G, Poland F, King M, et al. Community occupational therapy for people with dementia and family carers (COTiD-UK) versus treatment as usual (valuing active life in dementia [VALID] programme): study protocol for a randomised controlled trial. Trials. 2016;17:65.
47. Kalia LV, Lang AE. Parkinson's disease. Lancet. 2015;386(9996):896–912.
48. Dorsey ER, Bloem BR. The Parkinson pandemic-a call to action. JAMA Neurol. 2018;75(1):9–10.
49. Sturkenboom IHWM, Thijssen MCE, Gons-van Elsacker JJ, Jansen IJH, Maasdam A, Schulten M, et al. Ergotherapie bij de ziekte van Parkinson, een richtlijn van Ergotherapie Nederland. Utrecht/Den Haag: Ergotherapie Nederland/Uitgeverij Lemma; 2008. [in Dutch].
50. Sturkenboom IHWM, Thijssen MCE, Gons-van Elsacker JJ, Jansen IJH, Maasdam A, Schulten M, et al. Guidelines for occupational therapy in Parkinson's disease rehabilitation. Nijmegen/ Miami: ParkinsonNet/NPF; 2011. http://parkinsonnet.info/guidelines. Accessed 10 Dec 2019.
51. Sturkenboom IH, Graff MJ, Hendriks JC, Veenhuizen Y, Munneke M, Bloem BR, et al. Efficacy of occupational therapy for patients with Parkinson's disease: a randomised controlled trial. Lancet Neurol. 2014;13(6):557–66.

52. Sturkenboom IH, Nijhuis-van der Sanden MW, Graff MJ. A process evaluation of a home-based occupational therapy intervention for Parkinson's patients and their caregivers performed alongside a randomized controlled trial. Clin Rehabil. 2016;30(12):1186–99.
53. Law M, Baptiste S, Carswell A, McColl M, Polatajko H, Pollock N. Canadian occupational performance measure. Toronto: CAOT Publications; 2005.
54. Fisher AG. Assessment of motor and process skills: volume I-development, standardization, and administration manual. Fort Collins: Three Star Press; 2005.
55. Chapparo C, Ranka J. PRPP system of task analysis: user's training manual-research edition. Sydney: OP Network; 2012.
56. Law M, Cooper B, Strong S, Stewart D, Rigby P, Letts L. The person-environment-occupation model: a transactive approach to occupational performance. Can J Occup Ther. 1996;63(1):9–23.
57. Nonnekes J, Ruzicka E, Nieuwboer A, Hallett M, Fasano A, Bloem BR. Compensation strategies for gait impairments in Parkinson disease: a review. JAMA Neurol. 2019;76(6):718–25.
58. Bloem BR, Munneke M. Revolutionising management of chronic disease: the ParkinsonNet approach. BMJ. 2014;348:g1838.
59. Sturkenboom IHWM, Thijssen MCE, Gons-van Elsacker JJ, Jansen IJH, Maasdam A, Schulten M, et al. Linee guida per la Terapia Occupazionale nella Riabilitazione della Malattia di Parkinson [Guidelines for occupational therapy in Parkinson's disease rehabilitation]. Rome: SITO; 2016. http://www.parkinsonnet.info/guidelines. Accessed 10 Dec 2019.
60. Henry JD, von Hippel W, Thompson C, Pulford P, Sachdev P, Brodaty H. Social behavior in mild cognitive impairment and early dementia. J Clin Exp Neuropsychol. 2012;34(8):806–13.
61. Wilson RS, Krueger KR, Arnold SE, Schneider JA, Kelly JF, Barnes LL, et al. Loneliness and risk of Alzheimer disease. Arch Gen Psychiatry. 2007;64(2):234–40.
62. Barberger-Gateau P, Fabrigoule C, Amieva H, Helmer C, Dartigues JF. The disablement process: a conceptual framework for dementia-associated disability. Dement Geriatr Cogn Disord. 2002;13(2):60–6.
63. Sorensen LV, Waldorff FB, Waldemar G. Social participation in home-living patients with mild Alzheimer's disease. Arch Gerontol Geriatr. 2008;47(3):291–301.
64. Donkers HW, van der Veen DJ, Vernooij-Dassen MJ, Nijhuis-van der Sanden MWG, Graff MJL. Social participation of people with cognitive problems and their caregivers: a feasibility evaluation of the social fitness programme. Int J Geriatr Psychiatry. 2017;32(12):e50–63.
65. Samuelsson AM, Annerstedt L, Elmstahl S, Samuelsson S, Grafstrom M. Burden of responsibility experienced by family caregivers of elderly dementia sufferers: analyses of strain, feelings and coping strategies. Scand J Caring Sci. 2001;15:25–33.
66. Adelman RD, Tmanova LL, Delgado D, Dion S, Lachs MS. Caregiver burden: a clinical review. JAMA. 2014;311(10):1052–60.
67. Soderhamn U, Landmark B, Eriksen S, Soderhamn O. Participation in physical and social activities among home-dwelling persons with dementia - experiences of next of kin. Psychol Res Behav Manag. 2013;6:29–36.
68. Haaften-van Dijk AM. Social participation and quality of life in dementia: implementation and effects of interventions using participation as strategy to improve quality of life of people with dementia and their carers. Amsterdam: VU; 2016.
69. Swaffer K. Dementia: stigma, language, and dementia-friendly. Dementia. 2014;13(6):709–16.
70. Zaccaria D, Guaita A, Salvini Porro G, Vitali S, Possenti M, Trabucchi M, editors. Dementia friendly community: the Italian experience of Abbiategrasso. In: International conference of Alzheimer's disease international, Kyoto; 2017.
71. Lin SY. 'Dementia-friendly communities' and being dementia friendly in healthcare settings. Curr Opin Psychiatry. 2017;30(2):145–50.
72. Turner N, Morken L. Better together: a comparative analysis of age-friendly and dementia friendly communities. Washington, DC: AARP; 2016. https://www.aarp.org/livable-communities/network-age-friendly-communities/info-2016/dementia-friendly-communities.html. Accessed 12 Mar 2019.

Maud J. L. Graff PhD/OTR, Professor in Occupational Therapy at the Radboud University Medical Center; Donders Institute for Brain, Cognition and Behavior; Dept. of Rehabilitation and Scientific Institute for Quality of Healthcare Research, Nijmegen, The Netherlands. Global Expert, Lecturer and Researcher on Community Occupational Therapy in Dementia Programme Expert Centre.

Lucia Bergamini MD, Medical Doctor, Geriatrician at Center for Cognitive Disorders for Adults and Elderly Mirandola, Health Local Agency Modena, Italy. Special Care Unit for Dementia and Behavioural and Psychological Symptoms of Dementia, CISA Mirandola, Italy.

Mandy Chamberlain MOTR/L, Occupational Therapist and founder of SeniorsFlourish.com, a website dedicated to helping occupational therapy practitioners be the best they can be when working with older adults through continuing education, resources and support. Colorado, USA.

Ingrid H. W. M. Sturkenboom PhD, Occupational therapist and researcher at Radboud university medical center; Donders Institute for Brain, Cognition and Behavior, Dept. of Rehabilitation, Nijmegen, The Netherlands. Global Expert Occupational therapy at ParkinsonNet International; Radboud university medical center, Center of Excellence for Parkinson's disease and movement disorders.

Occupational Therapy in the Intensive Care Unit

4

Nathan E. Brummel, Evelyn A. Álvarez, Cheryl L. Esbrook, Matthew F. Mart, Maricel Garrido, and Eduardo Tobar

4.1   Introduction and Background

The world population is aging. By 2050, the number of older adults, those age 65 years or older, is expected to triple to 1.5 billion [1]. While high-income nations will be affected, the majority of this growth in older adults is expected to occur in low- and middle-income nations. Accompanying this shift in demographics are age- and lifestyle-related increases in the incidence of non-communicable chronic diseases such as cancer, heart disease, diabetes, and dementia [1].

These worldwide demographic and health trends will affect the number of patients who develop critical illness. The incidence of common causes for intensive care unit (ICU) admission such as sepsis (i.e., infection complicated by organ

N. E. Brummel (✉)
Division of Pulmonary, Critical Care, and Sleep Medicine, Department of Internal Medicine, The Ohio State University Wexner Medical Center, Columbus, OH, USA
e-mail: nathan.brummel@osumc.edu

E. A. Álvarez
School of Occupational Therapy, Health Sciences Faculty, University of Chile, Santiago, Chile
e-mail: evelyn.alvarez@ucentral.cl

C. L. Esbrook
Department of Therapy Services, University of Chicago, Chicago, IL, USA
e-mail: Cheryl.Esbrook@uchospitals.edu

M. F. Mart
Department of Medicine, Vanderbilt University Medical Center, Nashville, TN, USA
e-mail: matthew.f.mart@vumc.org

M. Garrido
Physical Medicine and Rehabilitation Service, University of Chile, Santiago, Chile

E. Tobar
Intensive Care Unit, Department of Internal Medicine, Clinical Hospital, University of Chile, Santiago, Chile
e-mail: etobar@hcuch.cl

© Springer Nature Switzerland AG 2020
C. Pozzi et al. (eds.), *Occupational Therapy for Older People*,
https://doi.org/10.1007/978-3-030-35731-3_4

failure), the acute respiratory distress syndrome (ARDS), and mechanical ventilation is greatest among those age 65 years or older [2–5]. Likewise, as the number persons with chronic diseases increases, and treatment for these conditions intensifies with advances in medicine, complications resulting in acute on chronic organ dysfunction necessitating ICU admission will also increase [6].

At present, an estimated 20 million people worldwide develop respiratory failure treated with mechanical ventilation each year. An equal proportion will develop sepsis (i.e., infections complicated by organ failure) [6]. Mortality from these causes of critical illness ranges from 10% to 40%. Thus, conservatively, over 12 million people survive a critical illness annually, a number that is expected to increase in coming years as continued advances in critical care result in further reductions in mortality from critical illness [7, 8].

In recent years, the critical care community has begun to broaden the lens through which critical care outcomes are viewed [9–11]. Whereas once short-term outcomes (eg., 28-day mortality, ventilator-free days) were the standard by which studies in critical illness were measured, studies describing the life-altering changes in function and ability to live independently suffered by survivors of critical illness have led the field to now consider the longer-term effects of critical illness. Two traditional main stays of caring for the critically ill patient, deep sedation and bed rest, have been shown to be associated with worse mortality, and among survivors, impairments in physical and cognitive function [12–15]. Interventions to reduce sedation and bed rest have been shown to reduce delirium during critical illness, and at hospital discharge, to reduce disability in activities of daily living (ADLs), improve muscle strength, and improve the ability to walk independently [16–21].

This chapter will describe the persistent impairments that affect a large number of survivors of critical illness using the World Health Organization's International Classification of Functionality, Disability, and Health (ICF) framework [22]. Then it will describe tools to assess cognitive and physical function in patients with critical illness. Finally, it will discuss the role of occupational therapy in today's modern ICUs where the aim is to keep patients awake, engaged, and moving.

4.2 Long-Term Outcomes After Critical Illness and Post-Intensive Care Syndrome

The first studies evaluating patients who survived critical illness were performed in those with ARDS in the 1970s [4, 5]. Nevertheless, it was only in the early 2000s when large cohort studies began to describe the high proportion of patients with long-term cognitive, physical, and mental health impairments and reduced quality of life that these issues came to the attention of the critical care research and clinical communities [23–30]. To increase awareness of these long-term adverse effects of critical illness experts in the field of post-critical illness outcomes proposed the term post-intensive care syndrome (PICS) [16, 30]. PICS is defined as new or worsened impairments in cognitive, physical, or mental health functioning that persist beyond hospital discharge. PICS is common among survivors of critical illness, with at least one impairment present in 60–80% of survivors 1 year after their illness [31].

Although the manifestations of PICS can be wide-ranging, the domains most closely aligned with the role of occupational therapy are cognitive and physical function.

Long-term cognitive impairment (LTCI) affects 50–70% of survivors of critical illness 1 year after discharge from the ICU and beyond [27, 32]. Multiple areas of cognition are affected, including memory, processing speed, global cognition, and executive function [33]. In one out of four survivors, these impairments can be as severe as Alzheimer's disease. Key risk factors during critical illness are not completely understood. Nevertheless, delirium, hypoxemia, hypoglycemia, metabolic disturbances, and psychoactive medications such as sedatives and opiates have been shown to be associated with long-term cognition in survivors [34].

Physical impairments in survivors of critical illness primarily take the form of neuromuscular weakness, commonly referred to as ICU-acquired weakness (ICUAW) [35]. ICUAW is a syndrome of generalized limb weakness that developed while the patient is critically ill and for which there is no alternative explanation other than the critical illness itself [35]. Neuromuscular weakness after critical illness can range in severity from minor weakness to complete paralysis [36]. Using a conservative definition of a score of <4 on the Medical Research Council muscle strength score (range 0–5, where higher scores indicate greater strength), recent clinical practice guidelines identified ICUAW in 33–50% of survivors of critical illness [37, 38]. Underlying mechanisms by which ICUAW develops are unclear, though important risk factors include age, duration of bed rest, ICU length of stay, and sedative medications [14, 15, 38, 39].

While scientific understanding of the cognitive and physical impairments in survivors of critical illness has grown in recent years, the underlying biological mechanisms and therefore interventions to alter the course of these impairments remain unclear. A number of factors contribute these gaps in knowledge. First, only 2% of all studies published in the critical care literature over the past 40 years have focused on outcomes in survivors of critical illness. Second, outcome assessment tools used in these studies are heterogenous [40]. For example, a recent scoping review identified 425 studies of cognitive, physical, and mental health outcomes in survivors of critical illness and reported that 250 different tools were used to assess outcomes [40]. Finally, significant gaps remain between outcomes considered important by patients and their families and those considered important by clinicians and researchers [41].

Therefore, due to the complexity and diversity of impairments present in survivors of critical illness existing operational frameworks can be applied to studies of survivors of critical illness as a means by which to clarify language surrounding outcomes of interest, increase understanding of multiple interrelated factors resulting in impairments in survivors of illness, and to place the study of long-term outcomes in patients with critical illness in the larger context of disability research.

4.3 The International Classification of Functionality, Disability, and Health (ICF)

In 2001, the World Health Organization approved the International Classification of Functionality, Disability and Health, a conceptual framework which describes how health conditions affect a person's function across multiple domains in the context of biopsychosocial and personal factors using a comprehensive, universal, and internationally accepted model and taxonomy [22]. This common model and language, therefore, provides a scientific basis for understanding and studying outcomes while also facilitating interprofessional communication across fields and levels of care. In addition, by incorporating factors external to one's disease, the ICF model changes the focus of disabilities as a problem of the person to disability as a neutral, socially created problem.

As with earlier models that classify function and disability, the ICF considers the effect of a health condition on organ systems and their function (body structures and function), the activities a person can perform under standard conditions (activity limitations), and what a person does in his or her usual environment (participation restrictions, Fig. 4.1). The ICF also integrates the context in which the anatomical and functional changes are occurring (environment) and the person's experience of disability (personal factors).

The specific definitions of each of the six ICF domains considered in the context of survivorship from critical illness are as follows:

1. *Health condition*: This domain describes diseases, disorders, and injuries which provide the context for understanding disability and functioning. For example, common causes of critical illness such as sepsis or ARDS.
2. *Body functions and structures*: This domain describes the anatomical and/or functional alterations that the patient presents with as a consequence of critical illness at the cellular, organ, and organ system level. Assessing body functions and structure is familiar to the interprofessional critical care team focused on diagnosing, treating, and managing the pathophysiology of critical illness. Examples of measurements of body function and structures include clinical exam findings, laboratory tests, and markers of organ dysfunction.
3. *Activity limitations*: This domain corresponds to the performance of evaluations under standardized conditions. Examples of measurements of activity limita-

Fig. 4.1 The international classification of function

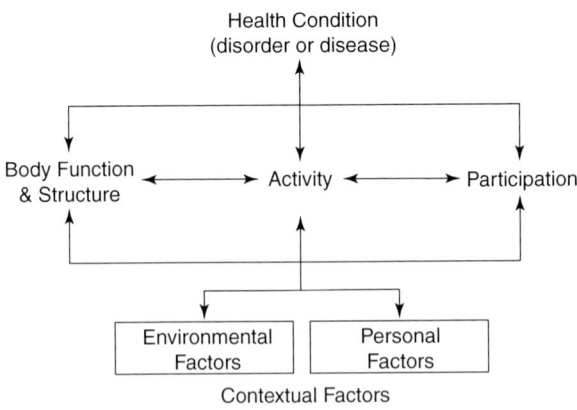

tions include a cognitive evaluation using an objective cognitive screening test such as the Montreal Cognitive Assessment (MoCA), an evaluation of exercise capacity using a 6-min walk test, or respiratory status using pulmonary function tests.

4. *Participation restriction*: This domain describes the interaction between a patient's functional limitations, expectations, and the social environment in which the patient lives and performs his or her daily activities. This domain includes activities such as those required to live independently (ie., basic and instrumental activities of daily living such as bathing, dressing, preparing a meal or managing finances) and other societal expectations such as employment.

5. *Environmental factors*: This domain includes social attitudes, characteristics of the built environment (e.g., accessible buildings and sidewalks), legal and social structures, and climate/terrain. For example, a survivor of sepsis with neuromuscular weakness and the inability to ambulate long distances may be unable to get to the store to shop for food independently because the neighborhood sidewalks lack cut-ins for her motorized scooter and therefore has a participation restriction. If her neighborhood made these changes to the built environment, she would no longer have this restriction.

6. *Personal factors*: This domain includes gender, age, coping styles, socioeconomic resources, behavior patterns, and other factors that influence how disability is experienced by the person. For example, a survivor of sepsis with a large family who lives close by and who has the financial means to afford in-home nursing care may be able to return home (rather than be discharged to a nursing home) following her hospitalization because of strong social support and socioeconomic resources.

4.4 The Role of Occupational Therapy in Critical Illness

Over the past two decades, critical care clinicians and researchers have begun to consider how traditional practices may lead to long-term complications of critical illness. Key modifiable risk factors for long-term cognitive impairment and ICUAW center around two common syndromes in patients with critical illness, delirium, and bed rest. Best clinical practices in the ICU now recommend that be managed with minimal or no sedation, leading to an increase in the number of alert patients [16, 42, 43]. Becuase patients are more alert, the modern ICU is a place where rehabilitation professionals such as occupational therapists (OTs) have assumed a more prominent and vital role in caring for previously comatose patients with critical illness.

In many ICUs worldwide, OTs work alongside physicians, nurses, pharmacists, respiratory therapists, physical therapists (PT), speech therapists, and social workers as part of a transdisciplinary team. Because each of these team members provides a unique skill, the OT's evaluation of the patient's health status and approach to management and treatment can play important roles in altering the course critical illness and its recovery.

4.4.1 Assessing the Patient with Critical Illness

By the very nature of critical illness and its treatment, patients in the ICU differ in important ways from those encountered in other inpatient and outpatient settings. Therefore, a unique set of assessment tools is needed to develop and carry out personalized recovery-focused plans across the continuum from acute critical illness to the months and years of survivorship that follow.

4.4.2 Pre-Illness Functional Status

Understanding a patient's pre-illness functional status (i.e., physical and cognitive) facilitates development of an individualized rehabilitation and treatment plan. During the very early stages of critical illness, however, the use of direct performance- and question-based measures may prove difficult due to factors related to the underlying critical illness and its treatment (e.g., endotracheal tubes, sedation, delirium, coma, muscle weakness). Thus, patient's family, friends, or caregivers serve as useful sources of information about a patient's pre-illness function.

4.4.3 Tools to Assess Pre-illness Cognitive Function

- *Informant Questionnaire on Cognitive Decline in the Elderly* is a 16-question survey of a patient's current cognitive function compared with 10 years ago [44, 45]. Surrogates rate patients on a 5-point scale ranging from "Much Improved" to "Much Worse.", where scores of 3 indicate no change. Scores on indivdual questions are divided by 16 to create a summary score. Higher scores indicate worsening of cognition.
- *Mini-Cog* is a brief, interactive, patient-only, three-item screening test for cognitive impairment. The patient is asked to immediately recall three items (i.e., banana, sunrise, and chair). The patient is then asked to draw a clock face indicating that the time is 10 after 11. After drawing the clock, the patient is asked to recall the three items.

4.4.4 Tools to Assess Pre-illness Disability

- *Barthel Index* is a ten-question survey of basic activities of daily living (BADLs) including feeding, bathing, grooming, dressing, bowels, bladder, toilet use, mobility on level surfaces and stairs [46]. The surrogate is asked whether the patient is independent or requires help. Scores range from 0 to 100, with lower scores indicating more severe disability in BADLs.
- *Functional Activities Questionnaire* is a ten-question survey of instrumental activities of daily living (IADLs) including paying bills, shopping, playing a game of skill, cooking, keeping track of current events, remembering appointments and family occasions, and traveling outside of one's neighborhood [47].

Scores range from 0 to 30, with higher scores indicating more severe disability in IADLs.

4.4.5 Functional Status During Critical Illness

During the acute phase of critical illness, both cognitive and physical function can change rapidly owing to the critical illness, its treatment, and related symptoms (e.g., pain and agitation); therefore, frequent assessment is needed. The following tools have therefore been developed and validated to assess the interrelated symptoms of pain, agitation, delirium, and weakness and the ability to carry out activities of daily living and mobility in patients with critical illness.

4.4.5.1 Pain Assessment
In patients who are awake and alert, the numeric rating scale (NRS) and visual analog scales can be used to assess pain. These scales ranging from 1 to 10 are commonly used outside of the ICU, and higher scores represent greater pain. In intubated and sedated patients, non-verbal cues and patient behaviors can be used to assess pain.

Behavioral Pain Scale (BPS) assesses facial expression, upper limb movement, and compliance with mechanical ventilation for indicators of pain [48]. Each behavior is scored from 1 to 4, with higher scores indicating more severe pain.

Critical Care Pain Observation Tool (CPOT) assesses facial expressions, body movements, muscle tension, and compliance with ventilation for intubated patients (or vocalization for patients who are not intubated) [49]. Each item is scored from 0 to 2, with higher scores representing greater pain.

4.4.5.2 Level of Consciousness Assessment
Richmond Agitation-Sedation Scale (RASS) is a 10-point scale used to measure level of consciousness using observation, physical, and verbal stimuli [50]. Scores range from −5 to +4. Negative scores represent depressed consciousness, 0 represents an alert and calm mental state, and positive scores represent agitation.

Riker Sedation-Agitation Scale (SAS) is a 7-point scale used to measure level of consciousness [51]. Scores from 1 to 3 represent depressed consciousness, a score of 4 represents a calm and cooperative patient, scores of 5–7 represent agitation.

4.4.5.3 Delirium Assessment
Confusion Assessment Method for the Intensive Care Unit (CAM-ICU) is a categorical delirium screening tool that, during a 1–2 min assessment, evaluates for four key features of delirium: (1) acute change or fluctuation in mental status, (2) inattention, (3) altered level of consciousness, and (4) disorganized thinking [52]. The CAM-ICU is positive, and delirium is considered present if the patient exhibits features 1, 2 and either feature 3 or feature 4. The CAM-ICU has been translated into over 30 languages.

Intensive Care Unit Delirium Screening Checklist (ICDSC) is a dimensional delirium screening tool where eight delirium symptoms are assessed over the course of 8–24 hours [53]. The presence of each of the following symptoms is given 1 point and a score of 4 or more indicates delirium: (1) altered level of consciousness, (2) inattention, (3) disorientation, (4) hallucinations, delusions, or psychosis, (5) psychomotor agitation or retardation, (6) inappropriate speech or mood, (7) sleep/wake disturbances, and (8) fluctuation of symptoms. Scores of 4 or greater represent delirium, and scores of 1–3 represent subsyndromal delirium.

4.4.5.4 Physical Function Assessment

Functional Status Score for the Intensive Care Unit (FSS-ICU) assesses while performing five tasks: rolling, transferring from supine to sitting, sitting at the edge of the bed, transferring from sitting to standing, and walking [54] using an eight-point ordinal scale ranging from 0 (unable to perform) to 7 (complete independence). Score range from 0 to 35, with higher scores indicating better physical function.

Physical Function ICU Test (PFIT) is a measure of strength and function. Patients are scored on their need for assistance moving from sit to stand (scored 0–2 according to the number of people needed), cadence while marching on the spot (scored as the number of steps/min), shoulder flexion and knee extension (scored 0 [no contraction] to 5 [movement against full gravity with resistance]) [55].

ICU Mobility Scale (IMS) is a structured method for quantifying mobility milestones [56]. Patients are scored daily on an 11-point ordinal scale ranging from 0 (lying in bed/passive exercises) to 10 (ambulating independently).

Medical Research Council (MRC) score is a manual test of muscle strength. Scores range from 0 (no contraction) to 5 (normal muscle strength) for six muscle groups (shoulder abduction, elbow flexion, wrist extension, hip flexion, knee extension, and ankle dorsiflexion) scored bilaterally [57]. Higher scores indicate better muscle strength. An MRC score of <48 has been used to define clinically significant ICUAW [37].

Handgrip Dynamometry is an objective method of volitional muscle force measurement. To accurately perform this evaluation, patients need an MRC score of 3 or higher in both elbow flexion and wrist extension. Patients should be seated as upright as possible (e.g., 70° to 90° from horizontal) and perform three trials sustained for at least 5–6 seconds. The values from the dynamometer can be compared with age- and sex-specific cut-offs to determine the presence of muscle weakness.

Hand-Held Dynamometry is an objective measure of major muscle groups (i.e., shoulder abduction, elbow flexion, wrist extension, hip flexion, knee extension, and ankle dorsiflexion). MRC scores of 3 or greater for the muscle group of interest and proper positioning of both the patient and the dynamometer are required to ensure accurate testing. As with the handgrip dynamometer, age- and sex-specific values can be used to determine the presences of muscle weakness.

Range of Motion (ROM) can be measured using a goniometer according to standard technique for all major joints: shoulder, elbow, wrist, hip, knee, and ankle. In the era before early mobility and rehabilitation, over one-third of patients with a prolonged stay in the ICU (e.g., 8 weeks or longer) developed significant joint contractures [58, 59]. Patient values can be compared with standard values for each joint to determine the presences of limitations in range of motion.

4.4.5.5 Assessing Activities of Daily Living

Functional Independence Measure (FIM) is a 16-item detailed, performance-based assessment of BADLs and cognition. It is divided into a motor score (grooming, bathing, upper body dressing, lower body dressing, toileting, bowel management, bladder management, bed to chair transfer, toilet transfer, shower transfer, locomotion [ambulatory or wheelchair level], climbing stairs) and a cognitive score (comprehension, expression, social interaction, problem solving, and memory) [60]. All assessments are scored from 1 to 7, with higher scores representing better function. The performance-based FIM may provide greater insight into a patient's ability to function independently while in the hospital than the questionnaire-based Barthel Index and FAQ described in the pre-hospital section.

4.5 OT-Directed Interventions to Reduce Delirium

Delirium is an acute confusional state characterized by inattention that affects up to half of patients with critical illness [61, 62]. The number of days of delirium are associated with worse cognitive function and disability among survivors [27, 63]. Multiple negative pharmacologic trials have renewed emphasis on non-pharmacologic interventions to reduce the delirium-related burden of suffering [64–66]. Existing non-pharmacologic interventions are characterized by nursing-driven interventions. Nevertheless, emerging data suggest that OT-specific interventions may also be helpful in reducing delirium [67].

The authors of this chapter randomized patients with critical illness to a non-pharmacologic delirium prevention protocol alone or a non-pharmacologic delirium prevention protocol plus a twice-daily, early and intensive, OT-specific protocol. The non-pharmacologic delirium prevention protocol consisted of reorientation, early mobilization, correction of sensory deficits, environmental modification (e.g., avoiding restraints, large clocks, and calendars), a sleep enhancement protocol, and avoidance of psychoactive medications. The OT-specific intervention (described below and in Table 4.1) was delivered for 40 min twice per day for up to 5 days beginning within 24 hours of ICU admission.

The OT-specific protocol (see Table 4.1) included the following:

1. *Polysensory stimulation* with items of different textures, smells, odors, sounds, tastes, or movements to increase a patient's level of alertness.
2. *Positioning* with devices and other adaptations to prevent edema and bedsores.
3. *Cognitive stimulation* consisting of exercises to activate mental functions including alertness, visual perception, memory, processing speed, problem solving, praxis, and language. Patients are given notebooks or electronic devices to perform these cognitive exercises. In addition, they are provided with playing cards, dominoes, memory games, and visuospatial construction games.
4. *Basic activities of daily living training* consisting of activities either simulating or performing actual BADLs (e.g., hygiene, grooming, eating).

Table 4.1 Example OT-directed intervention for delirium reduction

Intervention area	Activities	Device	Picture
Polysensory stimulation	Sensorial and motor stimulus	Things with different textures Different odors Different sounds Different movements	
Positioning and orthosis	Supine position Prone position Lateral recumbent Sitting Sitting on the edge of the bed Sitting on wheelchair	Splints Anti-edema wedge Ankle foot orthosis prevent bed Foot pillows	
Cognitive stimulation	Alertness Orientation Visual perception Memory Calculus Problem solving Praxis Language	Electronic tablet device Boards games Communication boards Augmentative and alternative communication devices	
Activities of daily living	Eating Grooming Dressing Bathing Toileting	Bathing and dressing aids Commodes Toilet aids Hand holding eating Special cutlery Special handle Sock aids Stocking aids Dressing sticks	

Upper extremity exercises	Hand exercisers Thumb and finger exercisers	Resistance bands Putty Egg shaped grip trainer Graded pinch
Family engagement	Education Family training	Brochures

Early mobilization	Active or active-assisted range of motion
	Upper extremity motor function
	Functional mobility
	  Supine to sit
	  Transfers–sit to stand
	  Transfers to chair
	  Transfers to commode
	  Gait
		Cones
		Transfers board
		Transfer belt
		Patient-handling equipment
		Bed rope ladders
		Walking assist device

5. *Upper extremity exercises* including hand and arm exercises using resistance bands, thumb and finger exercises using putty, egg-shaped hand exercise balls, and graded pinch exercisers.

6. *Family visitation* was encouraged each day.

During the hospitalization, fewer patients in the group randomized to the OT-specific intervention group developed delirium as compared with those who were managed with usual care (2/70 [3%] vs. 14/70 [20%], p = 0.001). Among those who became delirious, those randomized to the OT intervention had a shorter duration. Moreover, patients randomized to the OT intervention had higher motor and cognitive scores on the Functional Independence Measure.

4.5.1 OT Interventions for Reducing Immobility

In the past decade numerous randomized controlled trials and case-control studies have demonstrated the feasibility and safety of mobilizing and performing rehabilitation, typically through the use of treatment teams consisting of OTs and PTs [19–21, 68]. When these interventions begin during the earliest days of critical illness (e.g., within 1–3 days), patients who are treated with early mobility and rehabilitation have better muscle strength and ability to ambulate independently at hospital discharge than those who treated with usual care (i.e., later and less mobility and rehabilitation) [19–21]. Moreover, early mobility and rehabilitation interventions improve other outcomes including reducing the number of days on mechanical ventilation, and in ICU, and increasing the number of days alive and out of the hospital [20].

While primarily undertaken to improve muscle function and to reduce physical impairments and disabilities, early mobility and rehabilitation may also have effects on acute brain dysfunction during critical illness. Two multicenter randomized trials, which paired early mobility (eg., within the first 2 days of ICU admission) and rehabilitation interventions with a specific sedation management strategy (i.e., turning off sedation each morning and allowing patients to wake-up but remain comfortable) found that those in the intervention groups had 2–3 fewer days of delirium compared with those randomized to usual care [17, 18]. In contrast, randomized trials which provided a greater dose of mobility and rehabilitation, but which began later (eg., 5–7 days after ICU admission) and did not include specific sedation management strategies, found no such reduction in delirium or longer-term outcomes [69, 70]. Thus, although further study is needed to evaluate which type of mobility and rehabilitation interventions are most efficacious and which supporting elements are necessary to support these interventions, these data suggest that multicomponent strategies, involving multiple members of the ICU team, are required.

In summary, current data on early mobility and rehabilitation indicate that these practices are feasible, safe, and effective in reducing the short-term physical and cognitive sequelae of critical illness. Based on these data, clinical practice guidelines endorsed by the Society of Critical Care Medicine, the United Kingdom's National Institute for Health Care and Excellence (NICE), the Brazilian Association of Intensive Care Medicine, for example, recommend that patients be managed with these strategies [19, 71, 72].

Despite the evidence that it can improve outcomes, because early mobilization and rehabilitation of critically ill patients represents a sharp departure from the traditional practices of deep sedation and bed rest, the following section describes useful tools which can be used by OTs (and other ICU clinicians) to increase mobility among patients with critical illness.

4.5.2 Assessing Safety for Early Mobility and Rehabilitation

Rehabilitation/early mobility are safe [68]. Two systematic reviews which included over 30,000 mobility session found adverse events to occur in fewer than 2% of sessions [19, 68]. Of these adverse events, clinically significant adverse events occur in <1%. The majority of these events were due to transient hypoxemia and hemodynamic instability. Generalized safety criteria for starting and stopping rehabilitation/early mobility were developed as part of the 2018 Pain, Agitation, Delirium, Immobility, and Sleep Disruption (PAIDS) guidelines (see Table 4.2) and serve as a useful starting point for implementing these interventions [19].

4.5.3 Early Mobility and Rehabilitation Protocols

A number of different early mobility and rehabilitation interventions have been studied [73]. Although these interventions differ in specific content, ICU settings, and patient populations, no clear interventional protocol has emerged. The most commonly studied type of interventions, however, are those using progressive mobility. The authors of this chapter have published studies using OT- and PT-based progressive mobility protocols and present the following as an example protocol (see Fig. 4.2) [17, 74–76].

4.5.4 Example Progressive Mobility Protocol

The goal of progressive mobility protocols is to advance patients from passive range of motion exercises along a series of more difficult exercises up to independent ambulation using a "Sit, Stand, then Walk" approach. Sessions can progress rapidly in functional patients, with the goal of having patients achieve his or her "maximal functional milestone" (see Fig. 4.2).

First, patients should be assessed for the presence of any safety criteria that would preclude safely performing mobility exercises (see Table 4.2). During the intervention, patients are monitored for the development of any stopping criteria (see Table 4.2). If stopping criteria develop, the mobility session should be halted and the patient placed in a resting position (e.g., seated in a chair, seated at the edge of the bed, or supine in bed). If the safety criteria resolve, the session may then proceed at the therapists' discretion.

Table 4.2 Safety criteria for starting and stopping early mobility in patients with critical illness [19]

System	Starting a rehabilitation/mobility session	Stopping a rehabilitation/mobility session
	Rehabilitation or mobility can be "started" when ALL of the following parameters are present	Rehabilitation or mobility should be "stopped" when ANY of the following parameters are present
Cardiovascular	• Heart rate is between 60 and 130 beats/min, • Systolic blood pressure is between 90 and 180 mmHg, or • Mean arterial pressure is between 60 and 100 mmHg	• Heart rate decreases below 60 or increases above 130 beats/min, • Systolic blood pressure decreases below 90 or increases above 180 mmHg, or • Mean arterial pressure decreases below 60 or increases above 100 mmHg
Respiratory	• Respiratory rate is between 5 and 40 breaths/min • $SpO_2 \geq 88\%$ • $FiO_2 < 0.6$ and positive end-expiratory pressure <10 • Airway (endotracheal tube or tracheostomy) is adequately secured	• Respiratory rate decreases below 5 or increases above 40 breaths per minute • SpO_2 decreases below 88% • Concerns regarding adequate securement of airway (endotracheal tube or tracheostomy)
Neurologic	• Able to open eyes to voice	• Changes in consciousness, such as not following directions, lightheadedness, combative or agitated
	In addition, the following clinical signs and symptoms should be "absent" • New or symptomatic arrhythmia • Chest pain with concern for myocardial ischemia • Unstable spinal injury or lesion • Unstable fracture • Active or uncontrolled gastrointestinal bleed	In addition, if the following clinical signs, symptoms or events develop and appear clinically relevant • New/symptomatic arrhythmia • Chest pain with concern for myocardial ischemia • Ventilator asynchrony • Fall • Bleeding • Medical device removal or malfunction • Distress reported by patient or observed by clinician
Other	Mobility sessions may be performed with the following • Femoral vascular access devices, with exception of femoral sheaths in which hip mobilization is generally avoided • During continuous renal replacement therapy • Infusion of vasoactive medications	

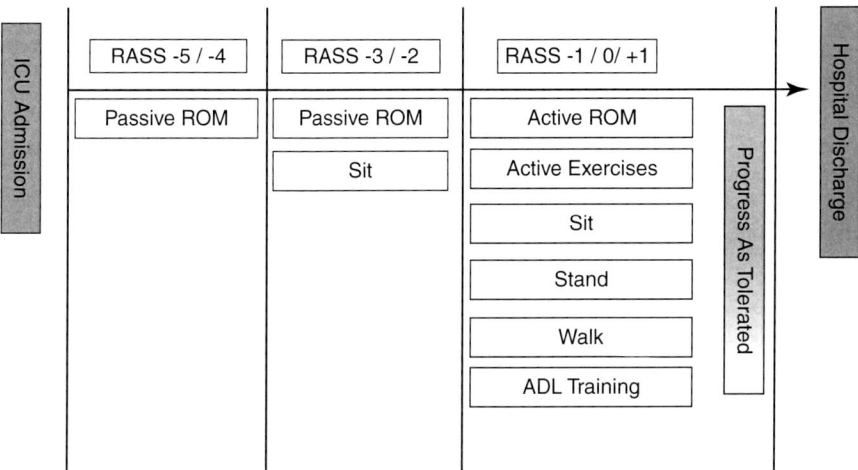

Fig. 4.2 Example progressive mobility protocol

The patient's level of consciousness can be used to guide which interventions can be delivered. Comatose patients (those with a RASS −5 or −4) are unable to participate in active interventions and therefore should be managed with passive range of motion of all major joints (e.g., extension and flexion of fingers, wrists, elbows, knees, and ankles; shoulder flexion; flexion, abduction, and adduction of hips; and ankle dorsiflexion and plantar flexion). Patients who open their eyes to voice (RASS −3 or −2), but who are unable to follow simple commands, can likewise undergo passive range of motion exercises. Occasionally, performing passive range of motion exercises may stimulate a patient to become more alert. If this is the case, the session can progress to the next level of exercises.

Awake and calm patients (RASS −1, 0, to +1) can perform a wider variety of rehabilitation/mobility interventions. Patients should begin with active, or active-assisted range of motion exercises of all major joints performed in the semirecumbent position. If able, the patient can then progress to bed mobility exercises (e.g., lateral rolling and supine to sit), dangling his or her feet at the edge of the bed, postural training, sitting balance exercises (such as reaching in and out of the base of support and challenges to elicit righting reflexes). While upright, the patient can undergo training in activities of daily living (eating or simulated eating, grooming, bathing, dressing, and toileting), in the sitting or standing position, as appropriate. Transfer training from the seated to standing position and from the bed to chair or commode can be performed, using multiple repetitions (and modifications of technique made). Standing exercises such as reaching in and out of the base of support, mini-squats, marching, and ambulation (with or without assist devices). Prior to performing standing exercises, the therapist should judge factors that could make standing unsafe (e.g., the patient's sitting balance, lower extremity strength, and the absence of impulsive behavior).

Throughout each session the therapist should educate the patient on energy conservation, work simplification, and breathing techniques which can increase overall activity tolerance.

4.6   Conclusion

The number of survivors of critical illness worldwide is increasing, but many are left with long-term impairments in cognition and physical function that affect the ability to function independently. Use of standard terminology and existing models such as the World Health Organization's International Classification of Functionality, Disability, and Health can be used to facilitate interprofessional communication. Delirium and bed rest are modifiable risk factors which are the focus of OT-driven interventions.

Key Messages

1. Post-intensive care syndrome (PICS) is defined as new or worsened impairments in cognitive, physical, or mental health functioning that persist beyond hospital discharge and is present in 60–80% of survivors 1 year after their illness.
2. The International Classification of Functionality, Disability and Health is a conceptual framework provides a scientific basis for understanding and studying outcomes while also facilitating interprofessional communication across fields and levels of care.
3. During acute critical illness cognitive and physical function changes rapidly owing to the critical illness, its treatment, and related symptoms (e.g., pain and agitation). Frequent assessment of function, using validated tools, is necessary.
4. Important modifiable risk factors for PICS include delirium and bed rest.
5. OT-directed interventions such as polysensory stimulation, cognitive stimulation, training in activities of daily living, and progressive mobility can be used to reduce delirium and bed rest, with the goal of improving long-term function in survivors.

References

1. National Institute on Aging. Global health and aging. Washington: Department of Health and Human Services. p. 2011.
2. Martin GS, Mannino DM, Eaton S, Moss M. The epidemiology of sepsis in the United States from 1979 through 2000. N Engl J Med. 2003;348:1546–54.
3. Martin GS, Mannino DM, Moss M. The effect of age on the development and outcome of adult sepsis. Crit Care Med. 2006;34:15–21.
4. Rubenfeld GD, Caldwell E, Peabody E, Weaver J, Martin DP, Neff M, Stern EJ, Hudson LD. Incidence and outcomes of acute lung injury. N Engl J Med. 2005;353:1685–93.

5. Needham DM, Bronskill SE, Sibbald WJ, Pronovost PJ, Laupacis A. Mechanical ventilation in Ontario, 1992-2000: incidence, survival, and hospital bed utilization of noncardiac surgery adult patients. Crit Care Med. 2004;32:1504–9.
6. Adhikari NK, Fowler RA, Bhagwanjee S, Rubenfeld GD. Critical care and the global burden of critical illness in adults. Lancet. 2010;376:1339–46.
7. Spragg RG, Bernard GR, Checkley W, Curtis JR, Gajic O, Guyatt G, Hall J, Israel E, Jain M, Needham DM, Randolph AG, Rubenfeld GD, Schoenfeld D, Thompson BT, Ware LB, Young D, Harabin AL. Beyond mortality: future clinical research in acute lung injury. Am J Respir Crit Care Med. 2010;181:1121–7.
8. Kaukonen KM, Bailey M, Suzuki S, Pilcher D, Bellomo R. Mortality related to severe sepsis and septic shock among critically ill patients in Australia and New Zealand, 2000-2012. JAMA. 2014;311:1308–16.
9. Iwashyna TJ. Survivorship will be the defining challenge of critical care in the 21st century. Ann Intern Med. 2010;153:204–5.
10. Iwashyna TJ, Speelmon EC. Advancing a third revolution in critical care. Am J Respir Crit Care Med. 2016;194:782–3.
11. Denehy L, Hough CL. Critical illness, disability, and the road home. Intensive Care Med. 2017;43:1881–3.
12. Shehabi Y, Bellomo R, Reade MC, Bailey M, Bass F, Howe B, McArthur C, Seppelt IM, Webb S, Weisbrodt L. Sedation practice in intensive care evaluation study I, group ACT. Early intensive care sedation predicts long-term mortality in ventilated critically ill patients. Am J Respir Crit Care Med. 2012;186:724–31.
13. Shehabi Y, Chan L, Kadiman S, Alias A, Ismail WN, Tan MA, Khoo TM, Ali SB, Saman MA, Shaltut A, Tan CC, Yong CY, Bailey M, Sedation Practice in Intensive care Evaluation Study Group Investigators. Sedation depth and long-term mortality in mechanically ventilated critically ill adults: a prospective longitudinal multicentre cohort study. Intensive Care Med. 2013;39:910–8.
14. Fan E, Dowdy DW, Colantuoni E, Mendez-Tellez PA, Sevransky JE, Shanholtz C, Himmelfarb CR, Desai SV, Ciesla N, Herridge MS, Pronovost PJ, Needham DM. Physical complications in acute lung injury survivors: a two-year longitudinal prospective study. Crit Care Med. 2014;42:849–59.
15. Pfoh ER, Wozniak AW, Colantuoni E, Dinglas VD, Mendez-Tellez PA, Shanholtz C, Ciesla ND, Pronovost PJ, Needham DM. Physical declines occurring after hospital discharge in ARDS survivors: a 5-year longitudinal study. Intensive Care Med. 2016;42:1557–66.
16. Girard TD, Kress JP, Fuchs BD, Thomason JW, Schweickert WD, Pun BT, Taichman DB, Dunn JG, Pohlman AS, Kinniry PA, Jackson JC, Canonico AE, Light RW, Shintani AK, Thompson JL, Gordon SM, Hall JB, Dittus RS, Bernard GR, Ely EW. Efficacy and safety of a paired sedation and ventilator weaning protocol for mechanically ventilated patients in intensive care (awakening and breathing controlled trial): a randomised controlled trial. Lancet. 2008;371:126–34.
17. Schweickert WD, Pohlman MC, Pohlman AS, Nigos C, Pawlik AJ, Esbrook CL, Spears L, Miller M, Franczyk M, Deprizio D, Schmidt GA, Bowman A, Barr R, McCallister KE, Hall JB, Kress JP. Early physical and occupational therapy in mechanically ventilated, critically ill patients: a randomised controlled trial. Lancet. 2009;373:1874–82.
18. Schaller SJ, Anstey M, Blobner M, Edrich T, Grabitz SD, Gradwohl-Matis I, Heim M, Houle T, Kurth T, Latronico N, Lee J, Meyer MJ, Peponis T, Talmor D, Velmahos GC, Waak K, Walz JM, Zafonte R, Eikermann M, International Early S-gMRI. Early, goal-directed mobilisation in the surgical intensive care unit: a randomised controlled trial. Lancet. 2016;388:1377–88.
19. Devlin JW, Skrobik Y, Gelinas C, Needham DM, Slooter AJC, Pandharipande PP, Watson PL, Weinhouse GL, Nunnally ME, Rochwerg B, Balas MC, van den Boogaard M, Bosma KJ, Brummel NE, Chanques G, Denehy L, Drouot X, Fraser GL, Harris JE, Joffe AM, Kho ME, Kress JP, Lanphere JA, McKinley S, Neufeld KJ, Pisani MA, Payen JF, Pun BT, Puntillo KA, Riker RR, Robinson BRH, Shehabi Y, Szumita PM, Winkelman C, Centofanti JE, Price C, Nikayin S, Misak CJ, Flood PD, Kiedrowski K, Alhazzani W. Clinical practice guidelines for

the prevention and management of pain, agitation/sedation, delirium, immobility, and sleep disruption in adult patients in the ICU. Crit Care Med. 2018;46:e825–73.

20. Tipping CJ, Harrold M, Holland A, Romero L, Nisbet T, Hodgson CL. The effects of active mobilisation and rehabilitation in ICU on mortality and function: a systematic review. Intensive Care Med. 2017;43:171–83.

21. Castro-Avila AC, Seron P, Fan E, Gaete M, Mickan S. Effect of early rehabilitation during intensive care unit stay on functional status: systematic review and meta-analysis. PLoS One. 2015;10:e0130722.

22. World Health Organization. Towards a common language for functioning, disability, and health. Geneva: WHO; 2002.

23. Herridge MS, Cheung AM, Tansey CM, Matte-Martyn A, Diaz-Granados N, Al-Saidi F, Cooper AB, Guest CB, Mazer CD, Mehta S, Stewart TE, Barr A, Cook D, Slutsky AS, Canadian Critical Care Trials Group. One-year outcomes in survivors of the acute respiratory distress syndrome. N Engl J Med. 2003;348:683–93.

24. Herridge MS, Tansey CM, Matte A, Tomlinson G, Diaz-Granados N, Cooper A, Guest CB, Mazer CD, Mehta S, Stewart TE, Kudlow P, Cook D, Slutsky AS, Cheung AM, Canadian Critical Care Trials Group. Functional disability 5 years after acute respiratory distress syndrome. N Engl J Med. 2011;364:1293–304.

25. Iwashyna TJ, Ely EW, Smith DM, Langa KM. Long-term cognitive impairment and functional disability among survivors of severe sepsis. JAMA. 2010;304:1787–94.

26. Needham DM, Dinglas VD, Bienvenu OJ, Colantuoni E, Wozniak AW, Rice TW, Hopkins RO, Network NNA. One year outcomes in patients with acute lung injury randomised to initial trophic or full enteral feeding: prospective follow-up of EDEN randomised trial. BMJ. 2013;346:f1532.

27. Pandharipande PP, Girard TD, Jackson JC, Morandi A, Thompson JL, Pun BT, Brummel NE, Hughes CG, Vasilevskis EE, Shintani AK, Moons KG, Geevarghese SK, Canonico A, Hopkins RO, Bernard GR, Dittus RS, Ely EW, Investigators B-IS. Long-term cognitive impairment after critical illness. N Engl J Med. 2013;369:1306–16.

28. Jackson JC, Pandharipande PP, Girard TD, Brummel NE, Thompson JL, Hughes CG, Pun BT, Vasilevskis EE, Morandi A, Shintani AK, Hopkins RO, Bernard GR, Dittus RS, Ely EW, Bringing to light the Risk Factors and Incidence of Neuropsychological dysfunction in ICU survivors. Depression, post-traumatic stress disorder, and functional disability in survivors of critical illness in the BRAIN-ICU study: a longitudinal cohort study. Lancet Respir Med. 2014;2:369–79.

29. Needham DM, Davidson J, Cohen H, Hopkins RO, Weinert C, Wunsch H, Zawistowski C, Bemis-Dougherty A, Berney SC, Bienvenu OJ, Brady SL, Brodsky MB, Denehy L, Elliott D, Flatley C, Harabin AL, Jones C, Louis D, Meltzer W, Muldoon SR, Palmer JB, Perme C, Robinson M, Schmidt DM, Scruth E, Spill GR, Storey CP, Render M, Votto J, Harvey MA. Improving long-term outcomes after discharge from intensive care unit: report from a stakeholders' conference. Crit Care Med. 2012;40:502–9.

30. Elliott D, Davidson JE, Harvey MA, Bemis-Dougherty A, Hopkins RO, Iwashyna TJ, Wagner J, Weinert C, Wunsch H, Bienvenu OJ, Black G, Brady S, Brodsky MB, Deutschman C, Doepp D, Flatley C, Fosnight S, Gittler M, Gomez BT, Hyzy R, Louis D, Mandel R, Maxwell C, Muldoon SR, Perme CS, Reilly C, Robinson MR, Rubin E, Schmidt DM, Schuller J, Scruth E, Siegal E, Spill GR, Sprenger S, Straumanis JP, Sutton P, Swoboda SM, Twaddle ML, Needham DM. Exploring the scope of post-intensive care syndrome therapy and care: engagement of non-critical care providers and survivors in a second stakeholders meeting. Crit Care Med. 2014;42:2518–26.

31. Marra A, Pandharipande PP, Girard TD, Patel MB, Hughes CG, Jackson JC, Thompson JL, Chandrasekhar R, Ely EW, Brummel NE. Co-occurrence of post-intensive care syndrome problems among 406 survivors of critical illness. Crit Care Med. 2018;46:1393–401.

32. Hopkins RO, Weaver LK, Pope D, Orme JF, Bigler ED, Larson LV. Neuropsychological sequelae and impaired health status in survivors of severe acute respiratory distress syndrome. Am J Respir Crit Care Med. 1999;160:50–6.

33. Hopkins RO, Jackson JC. Short- and long-term cognitive outcomes in intensive care unit survivors. Clin Chest Med. 2009;30:143–53, ix.
34. Hopkins RO, Jackson JC. Long-term neurocognitive function after critical illness. Chest. 2006;130:869–78.
35. Stevens RD, Marshall SA, Cornblath DR, Hoke A, Needham DM, de Jonghe B, Ali NA, Sharshar T. A framework for diagnosing and classifying intensive care unit-acquired weakness. Crit Care Med. 2009;37:S299–308.
36. Ali NA, O'Brien JM Jr, Hoffmann SP, Phillips G, Garland A, Finley JC, Almoosa K, Hejal R, Wolf KM, Lemeshow S, Connors AF Jr, Marsh CB, Midwest Critical Care C. Acquired weakness, handgrip strength, and mortality in critically ill patients. Am J Respir Crit Care Med. 2008;178:261–8.
37. Fan E, Cheek F, Chlan L, Gosselink R, Hart N, Herridge MS, Hopkins RO, Hough CL, Kress JP, Latronico N, Moss M, Needham DM, Rich MM, Stevens RD, Wilson KC, Winkelman C, Zochodne DW, Ali NA, ATSCoI-aWi A, American Thoracic S. An official American Thoracic Society Clinical Practice guideline: the diagnosis of intensive care unit-acquired weakness in adults. Am J Respir Crit Care Med. 2014;190:1437–46.
38. Kress JP, Hall JB. ICU-acquired weakness and recovery from critical illness. N Engl J Med. 2014;370:1626–35.
39. Puthucheary ZA, Rawal J, McPhail M, Connolly B, Ratnayake G, Chan P, Hopkinson NS, Phadke R, Dew T, Sidhu PS, Velloso C, Seymour J, Agley CC, Selby A, Limb M, Edwards LM, Smith K, Rowlerson A, Rennie MJ, Moxham J, Harridge SD, Hart N, Montgomery HE. Acute skeletal muscle wasting in critical illness. JAMA. 2013;310:1591–600.
40. Turnbull AE, Rabiee A, Davis WE, Nasser MF, Venna VR, Lolitha R, Hopkins RO, Bienvenu OJ, Robinson KA, Needham DM. Outcome measurement in ICU survivorship research from 1970 to 2013: a scoping review of 425 publications. Crit Care Med. 2016;44:1267–77.
41. Dinglas VD, Chessare CM, Davis WE, Parker A, Friedman LA, Colantuoni E, Bingham CO, Turnbull AE, Needham DM. Perspectives of survivors, families and researchers on key outcomes for research in acute respiratory failure. Thorax. 2018;73:7–12.
42. Kress JP, Pohlman AS, O'Connor MF, Hall JB. Daily interruption of sedative infusions in critically ill patients undergoing mechanical ventilation. N Engl J Med. 2000;342:1471–7.
43. Strom T, Martinussen T, Toft P. A protocol of no sedation for critically ill patients receiving mechanical ventilation: a randomised trial. Lancet. 2010;375:475–80.
44. Jorm AF, Christensen H, Henderson AS, Jacomb PA, Korten AE, Mackinnon A. Informant ratings of cognitive decline of elderly people: relationship to longitudinal change on cognitive tests. Age Ageing. 1996;25:125–9.
45. Borson S, Scanlan J, Brush M, Vitaliano P, Dokmak A. The mini-cog: a cognitive 'vital signs' measure for dementia screening in multi-lingual elderly. Int J Geriatr Psychiatry. 2000;15:1021–7.
46. Mahoney FI, Barthel DW. Functional evaluation: the Barthel index. Md State Med J. 1965;14:61–5.
47. Pfeffer RI, Kurosaki TT, Harrah CH Jr, Chance JM, Filos S. Measurement of functional activities in older adults in the community. J Gerontol. 1982;37:323–9.
48. Payen JF, Bru O, Bosson JL, Lagrasta A, Novel E, Deschaux I, Lavagne P, Jacquot C. Assessing pain in critically ill sedated patients by using a behavioral pain scale. Crit Care Med. 2001;29:2258–63.
49. Gelinas C, Johnston C. Pain assessment in the critically ill ventilated adult: validation of the critical-care pain observation tool and physiologic indicators. Clin J Pain. 2007;23:497–505.
50. Ely EW, Truman B, Shintani A, Thomason JW, Wheeler AP, Gordon S, Francis J, Speroff T, Gautam S, Margolin R, Sessler CN, Dittus RS, Bernard GR. Monitoring sedation status over time in ICU patients: reliability and validity of the Richmond agitation-sedation scale (RASS). JAMA. 2003;289:2983–91.
51. Riker RR, Picard JT, Fraser GL. Prospective evaluation of the sedation-agitation scale for adult critically ill patients. Crit Care Med. 1999;27:1325–9.

52. Ely EW, Inouye SK, Bernard GR, Gordon S, Francis J, May L, Truman B, Speroff T, Gautam S, Margolin R, Hart RP, Dittus R. Delirium in mechanically ventilated patients: validity and reliability of the confusion assessment method for the intensive care unit (CAM-ICU). JAMA. 2001;286:2703–10.

53. Bergeron N, Dubois MJ, Dumont M, Dial S, Skrobik Y. Intensive care delirium screening checklist: evaluation of a new screening tool. Intensive Care Med. 2001;27:859–64.

54. Zanni JM, Korupolu R, Fan E, Pradhan P, Janjua K, Palmer JB, Brower RG, Needham DM. Rehabilitation therapy and outcomes in acute respiratory failure: an observational pilot project. J Crit Care. 2010;25:254–62.

55. Denehy L, de Morton NA, Skinner EH, Edbrooke L, Haines K, Warrillow S, Berney S. A physical function test for use in the intensive care unit: validity, responsiveness, and predictive utility of the physical function ICU test (scored). Phys Ther. 2013;93:1636–45.

56. Hodgson C, Needham D, Haines K, Bailey M, Ward A, Harrold M, Young P, Zanni J, Buhr H, Higgins A, Presneill J, Berney S. Feasibility and inter-rater reliability of the ICU mobility scale. Heart Lung. 2014;43:19–24.

57. Vanpee G, Hermans G, Segers J, Gosselink R. Assessment of limb muscle strength in critically ill patients: a systematic review. Crit Care Med. 2014;42:701–11.

58. Clavet H, Hebert PC, Fergusson DA, Doucette S, Trudel G. Joint contractures in the intensive care unit: association with resource utilization and ambulatory status at discharge. Disabil Rehabil. 2011;33:105–12.

59. Clavet H, Hebert PC, Fergusson D, Doucette S, Trudel G. Joint contracture following prolonged stay in the intensive care unit. CMAJ. 2008;178:691–7.

60. Dodds TA, Martin DP, Stolov WC, Deyo RA. A validation of the functional independence measurement and its performance among rehabilitation inpatients. Arch Phys Med Rehabil. 1993;74:531–6.

61. American Psychiatric Association, DSM-5 Task Force. Diagnostic and statistical manual of mental disorders: DSM-5. Washington, DC: American Psychiatric Association; 2013.

62. Brummel NE, Girard TD. Preventing delirium in the intensive care unit. Crit Care Clin. 2013;29:51–65.

63. Girard TD, Jackson JC, Pandharipande PP, Pun BT, Thompson JL, Shintani AK, Gordon SM, Canonico AE, Dittus RS, Bernard GR, Ely EW. Delirium as a predictor of long-term cognitive impairment in survivors of critical illness. Crit Care Med. 2010;38:1513–20.

64. Girard TD, Pandharipande PP, Carson SS, Schmidt GA, Wright PE, Canonico AE, Pun BT, Thompson JL, Shintani AK, Meltzer HY, Bernard GR, Dittus RS, Ely EW, Investigators MT. Feasibility, efficacy, and safety of antipsychotics for intensive care unit delirium: the MIND randomized, placebo-controlled trial. Crit Care Med. 2010;38:428–37.

65. Girard TD, Exline MC, Carson SS, Hough CL, Rock P, Gong MN, Douglas IS, Malhotra A, Owens RL, Feinstein DJ, Khan B, Pisani MA, Hyzy RC, Schmidt GA, Schweickert WD, Hite RD, Bowton DL, Masica AL, Thompson JL, Chandrasekhar R, Pun BT, Strength C, Boehm LM, Jackson JC, Pandharipande PP, Brummel NE, Hughes CG, Patel MB, Stollings JL, Bernard GR, Dittus RS, Ely EW, for the MIND-USA Investigators. Haloperidol and ziprasidone for treatment of delirium in critical illness. N Engl J Med. 2018;379:2506–16.

66. Page VJ, Ely EW, Gates S, Zhao XB, Alce T, Shintani A, Jackson J, Perkins GD, McAuley DF. Effect of intravenous haloperidol on the duration of delirium and coma in critically ill patients (Hope-ICU): a randomised, double-blind, placebo-controlled trial. Lancet Respir Med. 2013;1:515–23.

67. Alvarez EA, Garrido MA, Tobar EA, Prieto SA, Vergara SO, Briceno CD, Gonzalez FJ. Occupational therapy for delirium management in elderly patients without mechanical ventilation in an intensive care unit: a pilot randomized clinical trial. J Crit Care. 2017;37:85–90.

68. Nydahl P, Sricharoenchai T, Chandra S, Kundt FS, Huang M, Fischill M, Needham DM. Safety of patient mobilization and rehabilitation in the intensive care unit. Systematic review with meta-analysis. Ann Am Thorac Soc. 2017;14:766–77.

69. Morris PE, Berry MJ, Files DC, Thompson JC, Hauser J, Flores L, Dhar S, Chmelo E, Lovato J, Case LD, Bakhru RN, Sarwal A, Parry SM, Campbell P, Mote A, Winkelman C,

Hite RD, Nicklas B, Chatterjee A, Young MP. Standardized rehabilitation and hospital length of stay among patients with acute respiratory failure: a randomized clinical trial. JAMA. 2016;315:2694–702.

70. Moss M, Nordon-Craft A, Malone D, Van Pelt D, Frankel SK, Warner ML, Kriekels W, McNulty M, Fairclough DL, Schenkman M. A randomized trial of an intensive physical therapy program for patients with acute respiratory failure. Am J Respir Crit Care Med. 2016;193:1101–10.

71. NICE CfCPa. Rehabilitation after critical illness. 2014 [cited 2016 February 8]. http://www.nice.org.uk/guidance/cg83.

72. Franca EE, Ferrari F, Fernandes P, Cavalcanti R, Duarte A, Martinez BP, Aquim EE, Damasceno MC. Physical therapy in critically ill adult patients: recommendations from the Brazilian Association of Intensive Care Medicine Department of Physical Therapy. Rev Bras Ter Intensiva. 2012;24:6–22.

73. Reid JC, Unger J, McCaskell D, Childerhose L, Zorko DJ, Kho ME. Physical rehabilitation interventions in the intensive care unit: a scoping review of 117 studies. J Intensive Care. 2018;6:80.

74. Pohlman MC, Schweickert WD, Pohlman AS, Nigos C, Pawlik AJ, Esbrook CL, Spears L, Miller M, Franczyk M, Deprizio D, Schmidt GA, Bowman A, Barr R, McCallister K, Hall JB, Kress JP. Feasibility of physical and occupational therapy beginning from initiation of mechanical ventilation. Crit Care Med. 2010;38:2089–94.

75. Brummel NE, Girard TD, Ely EW, Pandharipande PP, Morandi A, Hughes CG, Graves AJ, Shintani A, Murphy E, Work B, Pun BT, Boehm L, Gill TM, Dittus RS, Jackson JC. Feasibility and safety of early combined cognitive and physical therapy for critically ill medical and surgical patients: the Activity and Cognitive Therapy in ICU (ACT-ICU) trial. Intensive Care Med. 2014;40:370–9.

76. Brummel NE, Jackson JC, Girard TD, Pandharipande PP, Schiro E, Work B, Pun BT, Boehm L, Gill TM, Ely EW. A combined early cognitive and physical rehabilitation program for people who are critically ill: the activity and cognitive therapy in the intensive care unit (ACT-ICU) trial. Phys Ther. 2012;92:1580–92.

Occupational Therapy in Rehabilitation Settings

Alessandro Lanzoni, Elisabetta Romano,
Anette Hylen Ranhoff, Ellen Gjertsen Clark,
Morag Kelly Holter, and Charlotte Jørmeland

5.1   Introduction

The purpose of rehabilitation is to maximize function and minimize limitation of activity and restriction of participation resulting from an underlying impairment or disease [1]. Also for elderly people experiencing disease the aim of the rehabilitation process is to maximize their abilities and potential [2].

Making rehabilitation interventions tailored to the elderly person may be a challenge. This is due to the fact that the geriatric patient often has special needs associated with aging like cognitive impairment, comorbidities, polypharmacy, and end-of-life decisions. Every professional involved in geriatric rehabilitation should approach the patients being conscious of "frailty" that is a common geriatric syndrome. Clegg et al. defined "frailty" as "a state of vulnerability to poor resolution of homoeostasis after a stressor event and is a consequence of cumulative decline in many physiological systems during a lifetime" [3]. An effective rehabilitative intervention should include a proactive individualized assessment and care plan, which improves quality of life by reducing treatment burden, adverse events, and unplanned or uncoordinated care [4].

Geriatric rehabilitation can be defined as a multidisciplinary intervention aimed at older patients who are often frail and have comorbidities, including

A. Lanzoni (✉) · E. Romano
NODAIA Unit, Villa Igea Hospital, Modena, Italy

A. H. Ranhoff
Department of Clinical Science, University of Bergen, Bergen, Norway

Diakonhjemmet Hospital, Oslo, Norway
e-mail: anette.ranhoff@diakonsyk.no

E. G. Clark · M. K. Holter · C. Jørmeland
Diakonhjemmet Hospital, Oslo, Norway
e-mail: ellengjertsen.clark@diakonsyk.no; Morag.Holter@diakonsyk.no;
Charlotte.Jormeland@diakonsyk.no

© Springer Nature Switzerland AG 2020   77
C. Pozzi et al. (eds.), *Occupational Therapy for Older People*,
https://doi.org/10.1007/978-3-030-35731-3_5

cognitivevdysfunction and communication problems where the goal is to improve function and independence in performing activities [5].

Therefore, the challenge is to create a multidisciplinary intervention that activates different professions to respond to the different needs of the elderly.

5.2   Rehabilitation Settings

Rehabilitation can vary depending on the setting. Acute care, post-acute care, and community care should therefore be considered differently.

The initial acute care can start with an admission to a community and city hospital. In this initial phase it is essential that the elderly person is admitted to a separate unit in acute care hospital/medical center with a geriatric unit. But what could be defined as a "geriatric unit"? First of all, the team should have developed strong skills in managing geriatric clinical problems such as delirium, dementia, frailty, and malnutrition. All the members of the team should have specific professional skills with expertise in the geriatric field, such as treating geriatric patients with femur fracture while also having a broad geriatric competence including communicative skills for patients with cognitive impairment or caregivers with diverse problems [6]. Different approaches require different skills and must be considered in the professional training (see Chap. 8). High levels of managerial competence, flexibility, and empathy must also be strengthened.

The clinical aim in the acute care is clear. All the members of the team should have competence in essential elements of geriatric care such as frailty and comorbidity and complement each other's skill set.

For the post-acute care the rehabilitation process can continue in a geriatric rehabilitation facility. The rehabilitation can also continue in the community, for example, with the help of practitioners that can apply home interventions. Ideally, after an adequate assessment in the acute setting, it can be assumed that the appropriate setting for regaining participation and function should be in a rehabilitation unit. Bellelli et al. [7] underlined how it is mandatory to create an individualized and personalized rehabilitation path, or client-centered approach. Being able to make the rehabilitation pathway meaningful is a key factor in order to improve function and quality of life outcomes in older people with cognitive impairment. Indeed, a previous study showed how the increase of participation during rehabilitation sessions of occupational therapy and physiotherapy leads to better outcomes. Thus it is crucial to offer rehabilitation in a hospital specialized in geriatric rehabilitation where one also considers the occupational history of the person.

We know that every step in the rehabilitation process is important. Care transitions affect the caregivers in both a physical and social way, so inadequate transition can add to the caregiver's burden. It is also a risk for an early institutionalization of the geriatric patient. In light of this, to improve continuity and coordination of care in geriatric rehabilitation, an integrate care pathway has been developed and implemented in The Netherlands. The key points of this pathway are the presence of a coordinator, a triage instrument that instructs discharge nurses to gather information for potential patients for geriatric rehabilitation, the active involvement of patient and caregiver in every decisions, all patient discharge summaries (of all care professionals), and the meeting between care professionals of the various services [8]. The communication between different professionals could make the difference to avoid useless and harmful hospital admissions after a few days spent at home. It has been recognized [9] how polypharmacy, low functional status, and the long hospitalization in different settings could be risk factors for rapid re-admission. In these cases, the occupational therapist's expertise in the geriatric and psychogeriatric field can make the difference [10] in hospital care for people with severe cognitive impairment and delirium.

5.3 Rehabilitation of Geriatric People: The Role of the Occupational Therapist

Hospital admissions can often be linked to low levels of activity. With geriatric patients there is a higher risk of negative consequences, such as muscle weakness, contraction, and atrophy followed by decreased function and participation. This situation must be addressed by the personnel in charge of those patients in the Geriatric Rehabilitative Units before discharge [11]. Rehabilitation of geriatric patients has the potential to improve functional status, decrease permanent admissions to long-term care, and decrease mortality [1]. Occupational therapy has a unique role in rehabilitating older people with complex clinical situations by using a client-centered approach. This point of view has the potential to motivate the patients helping them to reach their goals. A successful rehabilitative alliance between the OT and the patient should recognize that the patient is the only real expert of his motivations, goals, and wishes. The therapist should avoid making decisions on his own or to "think for the patient" [12]. Occupational therapy process could also be conceived as a form of intervention to facilitate healthy aging through supporting social participation and addressing social isolation. This is a crucial factor to consider before planning discharge [13].

Giving for granted that early mobilization and stimulation of independency of the patients are provided as soon as possible, the occupational therapy process usually starts with the observation and analysis of participation of the patient while preserving the autonomy of the person. This could be carried out through informal observations, structured or semi-structured interviews such as Occupational Performance History Interview-II (OPHI-II) or Canadian Occupational Performance Measure (COPM) or through structured observations of performance by using standardized tools like—as an example—Assessment of Motor and Process Skills (AMPS), the ADL-focused Occupation-based Neurobehavioral Evaluation A-ONE, or the Perceive, Recall, Plan and Perform (PRPP).

Based on the cognitive function and ability to communicate an interview can be carried out with caregivers, but interviewing the patient directly is the gold-standard for client-centered intervention [14]. Complex, structured rehabilitative pathways could be feasible with a multidisciplinary approach. Improving communication, triage, and transfers of patients between the hospital, geriatric rehabilitation units, and primary care system are available organizational interventions to improve satisfaction of patients and caregivers [15].

5.4 Neurodegenerative Diseases and Complexity Factors

Neurodegenerative diseases are slowly progressing over months and year. Neurodegenerative diseases are generally affecting both physical and cognitive function.

5.4.1 Dementia

The most common dementia disorders are Alzheimer's disease (AD), Lewy body dementia (LBD), frontotemporal dementia (FTD), vascular dementia (VD); all with a common cognitive impairment such as lack of memory, poor executive functions, poor ability to understand abstraction and spatial deficiency. The different types of dementia have different symptom profiles and can include behavioral, physical, and emotional impairments. Rehabilitation in dementia is a topic of great relevance and growing interest today due to the reported low efficacy of drug therapies. Many interventions were born in the last decades and they are grouped with the name of "psycho-social interventions" or "non-pharmacological interventions." The rehabilitation of people with dementia is usually focused on maximizing the residual abilities rather than restoring lost functions and could be directed to the physical and social environmental factors known to affect the individual's ability for performing various activities. Formulating customized goals and interventions is crucial for people with dementia and their caregivers. To do so it is important to assess different domains through a comprehensive geriatric assessment (CGA) as described in Chap. 2 [4]. Implementing an extensive assessment is the first crucial step for delivering appropriate care. However, many types of dementia cannot be recognized at an early stage.

5.4.1.1 Assessment
Occupational therapy rehabilitation for people with dementia should focus on maximizing the preserved functions and participation in daily activities. To do so one must assess the needs and challenges experienced by the person with dementia. People with dementia experience problems in their activities of daily living at an early stage of the disease. An interview with the patient and/or the caregiver directed to understanding problems related to performing daily activities is useful at an early stage of the assessment. As was mentioned before, people with dementia should be interviewed by OT when possible.

An important thing to remember before providing an OT assessment is that people with dementia experience different realities which are often difficult and complex to understand. Assessments of the patient with dementia can help to understand their quality of life. However, it is important to gain an objective view and not only gather information from the caregiver as this will only paint a partial picture. An extensive assessment conducted by the OT should include an observation of the performance skills of the person in a familiar activity. This can be done by using standardized tools like the AMPS, A-ONE, PRPP or through observations based on specific assessments of models like occupational therapy intervention process model (OTIPM) and the model of human occupation (MOHO) to identify the patients' resources and shortcomings. Here we provide an example of an OT assessment.

Mr. P and the OT Assessment

Mr. P is an 86-year-old male with a suspected mild vascular dementia. He lives in a rural area but now he is in a hospital recovering after a traumatic injury. He has worked as a farmer before the retirement. He is married with two daughters. During an OT assessment Mr. P reveals that he misses a lot "doing his own business in the courtyard." The OT knew that his family had started to limit Mr. P's visit to the outside area in the last few weeks because they were worried about the risk of him falling which eventually happened inside the house. That leads to a sense of reported "unusefulness" by Mr. P. During the interview the OT recorded that Mr. P has always had a passion for taking care of the flowers and the plants. "Now I'm old" reports MR. P "but I have always been a great gardener! You know, it is important to care about your courtyard. It is like a business card of your family." The OT reports the thoughts of Mr. P in the occupational records and reflects on the impact of the physical and social environment on his quality of life.

After having illustrated the organization of the rehabilitation setting and how the occupational therapist can help the team in increasing the rehabilitation outcomes, in the next paragraph we will briefly clarify the different pathologies from a clinical point of view, showing the assessment and the various interventions of the occupational therapist.

5.4.1.2 Interventions Directed Toward ADL Independence

Usually, in mild dementia some individuals could benefit from strategy training intervention [16] but the vast majority of people should be approached in a compensatory way. Only a few persons with dementia are able to learn how to adapt their strategies to be more independent. In those cases the clinical experience suggests to start from their own coping solutions instead of teaching new ones.

Ms. L. and Strategy Training

Mr. L is a 76-year-old lady with a suspected diagnosis of mild dementia. She is now in a rehabilitative hospital recovering for hip replacement. Working with the OT, Mr. L improves performance and satisfactions in ADLs—especially dressing: this was possible due to an improvement of her own strategies. The OT observed how she applied spontaneously strategies for energy saving gathering all the dresses before wearing them. With the help of the OT she became aware of this action and they decided together to improve this technique: the dresses will be now put in front of her, on a chair, instead of on the bed on her side. In this way, it is easier for the lady to choose them correctly and after a few sessions she learns how to apply the new strategy consistently.

There is evidence supporting the benefits of occupation-based interventions and error-reduction learning to enhance occupational performance and delay functional decline in older adults with dementia [17]. Errorless learning is a common approach in practice: it is applied when people with dementia are enabled to perform activities in a setting that does not allow them to fail. When patients are encouraged to perform and in some way relearn meaningful activities in the early stages of their dementia, they may be enabled to increase their activity levels, boosting their sense of competence which could potentially lead to more independency and subsequently a better quality of life [18].

5.4.1.3 Behavioral and Psychological Symptoms

One of the most promising interventions for managing behavioral symptoms is the use of meaningful and/or graduated activities for people with dementia [19]. This approach is starting to be considered a standard approach to the problem even in national guidelines [20]. Redirecting the attention of people with dementia has shown to be an effective strategy to prevent and manage the BPSD. This usually also involves the use of effective communication and environmental strategies to increase the participation in activities. The OT plays a key role in this topic because of the professional unique understanding of activity analysis. OT should try to engage the people with dementia in meaningful activities with the involvement of the caregiver after an accurate multidomain assessment of the person. It can be beneficial if the communication or environmental tips are taught to the caregiver during the hospitalization in order to support the person with dementia after discharge. This could lead to a significant reduction of the frequency and severity of BPSD. The tailored activity program (TAP), for instance, could also be administered in clinical settings both to formal and informal caregivers [21].

5.4.2 Parkinson's Disease

Parkinson's disease (PD) is the second most common neuro-degenerative disorder. Different researches point the cause to the influence of a combination of environmental and genetic factors, [22] but it is clear that the degeneration continues over the years and involves both physical and cognitive function. The main motor symptoms of PD are bradykinesia, hypokinesia, rigidity, tremor, and disturbed posture reflexes which are often the medical focus in a clinical setting. However, the disability and difficulties performing daily activities affecting the quality of life are significantly influenced by non-motor manifestations like cognitive impairment, neuropsychiatric conditions, sleep, autonomic and sensory dysfunction, and fatigue [23].

The approach to the PD requires both pharmacological and non-pharmacological interventions. As the disease progresses, the effectiveness of the drugs is reduced. Over time the symptoms are more difficult to control with drugs and daily functioning and social participation are further compromised [24, 25]. Current evidence about the efficacy of occupational therapy intervention in PD is scarce, but the implication of occupational therapy in PD should encourage clients to engage an appropriate form of activity, enhance self-efficacy, and maintain participation in activity and roles [23]. In practice, the purpose of occupational therapy is to engage the person with PD in meaningful activities optimizing the activity performance and maintain the person's roles in his life context with the goal of improving function and quality of life [26].

It is necessary to assess the preserved abilities of the patient, the occupational performance as well as the physical and social environment. This will assist in determining intervention in order to reach the goals set by the patient and his/her caregiver.

5.4.2.1 Assessment

To follow the longitudinal course of Parkinson's disease the most used rating scale is the Unified Parkinson's Disease Rating Scale (UPDRS) that assesses three different sections (mentation, behavior, and mood; ADL; motor) by a medical interview (Table 5.1).

Table 5.1 Tools commonly used for the multidimensional assessment of patients with PD

Domain	Commonly used tools
Social status	Medical interview
Impairment and disability	Unified Parkinson's Disease Rating Scale (UPDRS) or Movement Disorder Society- Unified Parkinson's Disease Rating Scale (MDS-UPDRS)
Comorbidity	Cumulative Illness Rating Scale (CIRS)
Cognitive function	Mini Mental State Examination (MMSE)
Physical function	Timed Up and Go test (TUG), Tinetti scale
Functional status	Activities of Daily Living (ADL) and Instrumental Activities of Daily Living (IADL)
Psychological status	Beck Depression Inventory (BDI) or Geriatric Depression Scale (GDS)
Quality of life	Interviews or Parkinson's Disease Questionnaire (PDQ-39) or Parkinson's Disease Quality of Life Questionnaire (PDQL)
Global fatigue	Fatigue Severity Scale (FSS) or Modified Fatigue Impact Scale (MFIS)
Stage of Parkinson's disease	Hoehn and Yahr stage

Persons with PD often experience speech impairment, but where communication as well as the cognitive ability to answer direct questions about their personal point of view is preserved, interviews like Canadian Occupational Performance Measure (COPM) and Occupational Performance History Interview-II (OPHI-II) can be useful. These tools assess the participation in the activities and consider difficulties, needs, values, desires, requirements, and roles. In this way the patient is at the center of their own rehabilitation process. The crucial difference between these two tools and other standardized ADL questionnaires is the possibility of identifying the problems that the patient experiences as more significant. Especially the OPHI-II is a great tool to focus on the occupational identity of the patient.

It can also be useful to interview the caregiver by using the Canadian Occupational Performance Measure (COPM) or the ethnographic interview to identify the caregiver's experience and burden, physically and emotionally. After the interviews the OT should observe the patient in meaningful activities to assess the occupational performance. We recommend to observe skills in a familiar task and to use occupational therapy models and tools to guide the clinical reasoning.

5.4.2.2 Intervention
For patients at an early stage of the disease with minimal cognitive and/or motor limitations, the occupational therapy intervention focus can be to maintain and improve skills during the activity performance. However, in patients with more severe symptoms the approach has to be compensatory. From the perspective of a compensatory approach, the activities should be graduated and the physical and social environment modified in order to better support the patient's preserved abilities in the activity. Promoting participation in appropriate activities with tailored strategies can increase the quality of life of the patient. Occupational therapy can contribute to establish an appropriate routine, individualized cueing, and fatigue management techniques, apply a "single task" approach, and graduate the activity [27].

5.4.3   Delirium

Delirium is an acute brain dysfunction characterized by inattention and disturbance of awareness. It develops over a short period of time and can fluctuate during the course of the day; additional disturbances in cognition might be present [28]. As opposed to dementia the onset of delirium is acute. The literature agrees that a rapid intervention can reduce the duration of delirium and, consequently, the possible long-term sequelae [29]. A comprehensive treatment should be aimed at the specific symptoms of delirium and efforts to identify and treat the underlying causes. Recent studies have shown that occupational therapy can be useful for treating people with delirium [10, 30]. The focus should be on daily routines to promote structure and counteract occupational deprivation.

Table 5.2 Environmental factors in treating delirium

Environmental factors in treating delirium	Intervention/approach
Communication	Clear and concise information, repetition of information, information that will increase orientation
Orientation	Clocks and calendars
General care	Consistency in staff. Familiar faces, consistent routines
Senses	Make sure the patient has necessary aids: Clean glasses, hearing aid with batteries, dentures
Stimuli	Good lighting, reduction in noise, removal of any unnecessary objects although some personal and familiar objects can be a benefit
Family and carers	Involve family/carers who know and understand the patient's needs
Mobility	Patient should be up and moving regularly
ADL	Patient should be encouraged to be as independent in P-ADL. As possible

5.4.3.1 Assessment

The diagnosis of delirium could be demanding: symptoms of delirium might be mistaken for the fluctuation of cognitive function, or BPSD. Aside from the low levels of delirium detection in general [31, 32] it is currently unclear which assessment can be used in moderate to severe dementia patients and how accurately such tools could detect delirium [33]. However, health care providers should routinely use tools to detect delirium such as the 4AT [34] and confusion assessment method (CAM) [35] but there are also tools to detect changes in sedation status like the Richmond Agitation-Sedation Scale [36].

5.4.3.2 Intervention

There are many supportive and environmental measures delivered by a multidisciplinary team that can help the patient with delirium which will improve the outcome by limit risk factors [37]. Intervention should include re-orientation, early mobilization, nutrition, and sleep strategies. The aim is to increase orientation and limit stimuli which may cause stress and anxiety (Table 5.2).

Giving guidance to the patient's family and caregivers in using suitable communication is beneficial in order for them to care and promote the appropriate activities to help the individual. This also includes giving tips of how to keep the environment orderly and safe while decreasing the amount of unnecessary stimuli and at the same time encourage mobility and participation in meaningful activities [38].

5.5 Hip Fractures and Other Fragility Fractures

Hip fractures are common among older people, and the prognosis is serious in terms of mobility, independence in daily life activities, and cognition with 42% of patients never achieving the same function as before the fracture [39]. Hip fracture includes fractures in neck of femur, the trochanter region, and subtrochanter region of femur. Hip fracture patients are characterized by advanced age, frailty, comorbidity and many have cognitive impairment and dementia [40]. Hip fracture is the most serious fragility fracture, but also vertebral fractures, proximal humerus fractures, and wrist fractures are common in frail and multimorbid older people.

It is good evidence for interdisciplinary patient management through a clinical pathway from admission to discharge, and early mobilization and rehabilitation is strongly recommended [41].

The most important challenges in the rehabilitation after hip fracture are as follows:

- Mobility problems
- Balance problems, fall risk
- ADL-independency
- Cognitive impairment; chronic cognitive impairment (pre-fracture dementia) as well as acute cognitive impairment (delirium)
- Depressive symptoms and lack of motivation

5.5.1 Acute Stage of Orthogeriatrics

For an elderly person a fracture, caused by a fall or otherwise, can be both dramatic and traumatic [42, 43]. Along with the experience of pain at the time of the fracture and the operation there are always risks of further complications. A geriatric patient is particularly vulnerable in situations caused by fractures and they are more prone to develop infections and delirium. Post-operative treatment should be introduced immediately, including training with a view of regaining pre-fracture functions [44, 45]. Whereas the hospital admission should be facilitated as soon as possible discharge should be well planned, whether it is directed to a rehabilitation unit or directly to the patient's home [43]. Reasons for falls that may cause fractures are many and complicated. There are further needs for identifying them and to investigate how to reduce risks for new falls. Investigation of fall tendency in elderly patients needs a multidisciplinary approach and special competence in geriatrics, particularly for patients with many chronic syndromes and unclear reasons for fall [41]. The interdisciplinary team on the acute ward should include a specialist in orthopedics, a geriatrician, a nurse, a physiotherapist, and an occupational therapist. The OT is an essential part of the team in order to investigate how the patient's level of activity performance and function was before the fall. Furthermore it is important to collect information about the social and housing situation.

5.5.2 Assessment

Before setting goals for treatment it is important to identify the patients' physical and cognitive function before their fall. This can be achieved by interviewing the patient with either a semi-structured or a structured interview. As the patient is in a new situation and perhaps experiences this as a crisis, a semi-structured interview is

Table 5.3 Semi-structured interview if the caregiver answers replace "you" with "the patient"

Person	Activity	Environment home and social
What was the reason for admission to hospital?	*Mobility* do you use any walking aids?	Where do you live and with whom?
How and where did you fall?	Do you have any experiences of falling?	Do you live in an apartment or house?
What changes do you experience?	*B-ADL* do you need any help with dressing and bathing?	How is the access to your bathroom?
	I-ADL do you shop and cook for yourself?	What kind of help to you need?
	Do you organize your own economy?	Do you receive any help from the community or family?
	Do you use technical devices such as mobile phone, PC, etc.?	Do have stairs/steps/lift?
	Hobbies and interests	Do you have an aids/adaptions in the house?
	B-ADL do you need any help with dressing and bathing?	How is the access to your bathroom?
	I-ADL do you shop and cook by yourself?	What kind of help to you need?

often adequate. Many patients have cognitive impairment and therefore the caregiver may assist providing information about the premorbid levels of participation, in particular the level of mobility and independence in B-ADL and I-ADL. The interview should also address the patient's cognitive function (Table 5.3).

The information the team obtains about the patient's premorbid function can be a guideline to the level of rehabilitation. The patients who have been independent in self-care and mobility have better prognosis than those who are fragile and or have cognitive impairment [46]. At an early stage of the rehabilitation as the patient makes recovery and increases mobility it is important to observe the patient's motor and process skills during performance of an activity. Ideally a formal observation based tool should be used to assess these skills to perform B-ADL or I-ADL. Even if the observation is informal or not standardized the focus of the OT will be to identify critical performance skills for the patient and should include an evaluation of the patient's effort, efficiency, safety, and independence in performance of the occupation or activity. The findings are helpful in order to evaluate the level of rehabilitation needed or the amount of help the patient will need after discharge to his own home.

5.5.2.1 Intervention

Mobilization should commence within 24 h after surgery. The aim should be to sit out of bed within the first day and bear weight provided no restrictions are in place [47]. If necessary the patient should be helped to come up and sit on the side of the bed. The physiotherapist will encourage the patient to do exercises and teach them to use walking aids. The patient should be encouraged to be active in B-ADL right away. In order to facilitate for this the activity can be graded from lying in bed and washing the face and body, then sitting on the side of the bed, before gradually be independent in the bathroom with adaptions. Most commonly 3–5 days post-surgery the assessment of the patient's potential for rehabilitation is complete and a basic level of function is established. It is important to set goals for the rehabilitation as soon as possible, preferably by a client-centered interview like COPM. It is important that the goals for rehabilitation are meaningful for the patient in order to motivate them to be active in their own recovery.

The patient will continue training in mobility and should gradually become more independent performing B-ADL. In order to facilitate independent dressing, the patient should be encouraged to use easy dressing clothing items such as training trousers and tops and shoes with elastic laces or velcro. Patients should learn to dress the bad limb first and undress the good limb first.

Some patients may have restrictions in range of motion and may benefit from dressing aids such as dressing stick, long handled washing sponges, reacher, stocking aid long handled shoehorn (Table 5.4).

The occupational therapist has responsibility for adaption of aids along with the nurse and physiotherapists, and is central in the planning of discharge, especially when the patient is discharged straight home.

Mr. B.—An Orthogeriatric Case

When Mrs. B was admitted to the hospital with a hip fracture she was alert and coherently described the situation which led to her falling at home. Her daughter reported that the patient lived independently and took care of everything on her own, including shopping and paying her bills. The family had no concerns about Mrs. B's cognitive status nor her ability to live by herself. The OT assessed the patient during the morning ADL. Mrs. B needed some assistance getting out of bed, from there she was able to walk to the bathroom using the support of a tall walker. She washed and dressed her upper body independently while sitting down, but had difficulties washing and dressing her lower body. She expressed a desire to return home and continue to live there without any assistance. The OT and Mrs. B agreed to focus on how to become independent, keep her safe while getting dressed. During toilet visits they worked on the ability to stand and pull up her panties and pants without help. Then the next few mornings the OT taught the patient how to use a stocking puller and a reacher to put on her pants and socks. Before discharge the OT cooperated with the patient and her family to assess the home in order to provide necessary aids like a stool for the shower, an elevated toilet seat and gave advice on how to make some fall prevention and safety adaptions to the home.

5.5.2.2 Special Considerations

Many and varied factors may have a negative impact on the recovery after hip fracture in older adults.

Table 5.4 Example of dressing aids

Example of dressing aids	Uses
Long handled sponge	Washing feet
Dressing aid/reacher	Putting on trousers, aligning shoes
Stocking aid	Putting on socks and stockings
Shoehorn	Putting on shoes
Button hook	To help to button shirts

Depression Depressive symptoms are quite common in hip fracture patients, according to Lenze et al. [48] as many as 48% have significant depressive symptoms [43, 49]. Depression is not a normal symptom of aging, thus patients who lack motivation for treatment should be taken seriously as it could be a sign of depression. This will inhibit recovery and the potential for rehabilitation.

Cognitive Impairment Almost 40% of patients admitted to hospital because of hip fracture have underlying cognitive impairment. Cognitive impairment is associated with poor functional recovery, longer stay in hospital, and risk of institutionalization [43, 44]. However, patients with dementia who are recovering from hip fracture can still benefit from rehabilitation [50]. Consideration to the patient's cognitive impairment should be taken into account, for example, will the patient need simple instructions and an environment that does not cause anxiety. Patients with dementia are often frail and at great risk of developing delirium.

Delirium Many frail patients with cognitive impairment may develop delirium either pre-operatively or within the first post-operative days [44]. Patients should be clinically observed and routinely screened with 4AT before and post-surgery. Patients with delirium experience alterations of attention, they may have either higher or lower level of consciousness (hypoactive- or hyperactive-delirium). Commonly there are observed impairment of orientation, memory, and/or language [51].

5.5.2.3 Discharge

By the time the patients are expected to return home, they should be sufficiently mobile so that they can walk around safely in the home, with or without walking aids. The patients should be able to rise from chairs/beds in order to walk independently to the bathroom and use the toilet independently. They may need adaptions at home or simple aids to facilitate independence and safety. It is recommended with a home visit by an OT to both to assess the needs for aids and adaptions in relation to fall prevention [41]. Preferably this should take place before the patient is discharged. There are many things to be looked at and the focus is to eliminate hazards such as loose carpets and electric wires as well as challenging access with steps and stairs. Kitchen and bathroom cupboards should be arranged to reduce the need to bend, reach, or climb to access frequently used items. The bathroom may need adaptions for safe access to the toilet and shower and prevent danger of slipping. Older people have reduced eyesight and good lighting and should be recommended.

Reduced hearing can also be a hazard for the older person as they can get startled and fall [50]. If a preexisting dementia was present there may be a need for alarm, safety aids for the cooker and other electrical appliances, and for assistive technology. Many elderly people will be scared of falling again. It is thus important to encourage them to be active by providing the proper aids or amendments in their environment.

5.6 Stroke and Traumatic Brain Injury

Stroke includes cerebral infarction (85%) and bleeding (15%). Symptoms and functional problems are decided by the size of the damage on brain tissue, the location, and the pre-fracture status of the brain (aging and previous vascular and other pathology). Modern stroke care has contributed to better outcomes in patients. The care principles in the stroke-unit are interdisciplinary patient management for optimization of physiology to minimize brain injury and early mobilization and rehabilitation. The most common brain injury is subdural hematoma, followed by other traumatic hematoma (epidural, subarachnoidal, and intracerebral) often combined with contusion injuries and skull fractures. After the clinical situation is stabilized, these patients have many of the same problems and need the same rehabilitation as stroke patients.

A comprehensive assessment of medical issues, neurological deficits, physical and cognitive function, and ADL function is needed. The most important challenges in the rehabilitation after stroke and traumatic brain injury are the neurological deficits which are causing mobility problems, cognitive impairment, fatigue, depressive symptoms, decreased ADL-independency. All patients admitted to the hospital with a confirmed or suspected stroke should be admitted to a specialized stroke ward and referred for an assessment by all the professions in the interdisciplinary team, particularly the OT and PT. The assessments are crucial in order to consider the treatment plan and the need for rehabilitation. Intervention and assessment are both a continuous and interwoven process and will be reflected by the ongoing clinical reasoning by the OT. Early mobilization and task related training is a key factor and should be initiated as soon as the patient is medically stable, preferably within the first 24–48 h [52]. At an early stage the aim is usually to regain function before looking at compensatory interventions. It is a particular challenge within geriatrics to reveal new versus established outcomes as well as the different neurological outcomes versus normal changes due to aging for the respective age group [53].

5.6.1 Assessment

Occupational therapists have an important role in assessing cognitive outcomes and how it affects their performance in activity. A semi-structured interview in the initial stage will give an impression of how the patient can communicate and give relevant information of their situation and earlier level of function and participation. The first assessment is based on observation in a basic activity like grooming or eating. The OT will also obtain an impression of the patient s' resources and coping strategies. Even though the therapist does not hold a certification in the standardized and validated activity based assessments (e.g., AMPS, A-ONE, or PRPP), less structured observations of activity performance in meaningful activities may be accomplished. This may be very useful if the therapist stays focused assessing motor and processing skills as well as their communication skills during activity performance. It is important to grade and adapt the activities in order for the patient to achieve some sense of dignity and self-efficacy.

In most cases a combination of tests and observations in activities are used, often serving as a dual function of assessment and early rehabilitation. In many cases a systematic cognitive screening is conducted with tasks assessing memory, attention, visuo-spatial orientation, awareness of time and place, oral and written communication, apraxia, neglect, hearing and visual outcomes. This can be done with validated tools for desktop screening like LOTCA, MoCA, and trail making test. The combination of observing and analyzing the performance in an activity and the use of standardized tests may be useful and complement each other in the assessment. They may also indicate an area for further investigation. Each patient is unique and thus will experience a variance of outcomes and challenges (Table 5.5).

If the patient cannot communicate reliably information about the premorbid function must be obtained from others, for instance, next of kin. In the case of dysphagia, aphasia, or other language outcomes it is important to refer to a speech therapist as early as possible in order to draw the correct conclusions regarding potential cognitive outcomes.

Table 5.5 Outcomes commonly assessed in patients with stroke

Motor and sensibility functions	Vision and cognitive functions	Language and communication
• Sensibility (temperature, touch, location, kinetic/joint, stereognosis) • Strength/active function • Tonus • Tempo • Coordination • Fine motor skills • Balance (sitting and standing) • Mobility • Walking/gait • Fatigue • Edema • Pain	• Field of view • Motion of the eyes • Diplopia • Hearing • Spatial orientation • Attention/concentration • Memory • Agnosia (visual, tactile auditive) • Apraxia • Orientation (time, place, situation, community) • Neglect and idea of body • Judgment/impulse control • Insight • Executive functions (problem solving, abstract thinking, etc.) • Mood/psychological	• Aphasia (expressive/ impressive input/ output) • Dysarthria • Modulation of voice • Dysphagia (swallowing) • Articulation • Motion of lips and tongue • Speech apraxia

Mr. L—A Neurogeriatrics Case

Mrs. L has suffered a stroke and during the first assessment on the acute stroke ward the OT enters with the PT to find the patient laying on an angle in her bed. She can move her left leg slightly when asked, but not her left arm. The OT and PT work together with Mrs. L to mobilize her to the bedside. She tends to lean to her left and needs support by a person sitting on her left side in order to keep her balance while sitting. She has difficulty locating objects on her left, even when encouraged to look to her left. The PT finds that Mrs. L has decreased sensibility in her left leg, but can discriminate touch on her leg but she registers only pain stimuli on her left arm. She has slight movement in her left shoulder, but no active movement in her left arm or hand. When the OT assesses her eye motility she manages to move her eyes to the left, but her gaze drifts quickly to the center or to her right. In conversation Mrs. L talks about going home soon, seemingly unfaced with her inability to walk or use her left arm.

Due to her significant physical outcomes the OT plans her ADL observation the following day with the nurse in order to make it safe for all parties. They help the patient to the bedside where the nurse sits to the left while the OT has provided a washing basin, a cloth, and towel on the bedside table in front of the patient, the towel and cloth placed slightly to the left to stimulate attention to her left. During the activity the OT observes that Mrs. L has problems locating things to her left, she manages to undress her left sleeve without being prompted to do so. She makes no effort to include her left arm while washing and dressing and needs physical assistance to wash her right side. There is a delay in her asking for help when needed.

This initial assessment indicates intervention with focus on increased attention to the left, physical guiding of the left arm during activities (particularly meals, grooming, and dressing). Hopefully this will in time generate some insight for the patient and furthermore help in setting goals for rehabilitation.

5.6.2   Intervention

Setting goals for intervention must be client centered and based on their premorbid function. As the onset is acute and the patient may not fully understand the extent of their outcomes the OT may assist in setting realistic goals. The focus on client-centered approach may be challenging when the patients have difficulties expressing themselves due to communication problems or cognitive outcomes. In some cases the involvement of next of kin is then very beneficial.

5.6.2.1 Patients with Minimal Outcomes

Patients with smaller brain injury or strokes may be independent in mobilization and B-ADL within a few days and often have an early discharge. Patients with subtle outcomes or minimal cognitive challenges may not show difficulties performing activities in the confined setting of a hospital ward, but might experience problems in their daily activities later [54]. I-ADL activities are more complex and challenging in different environments and contexts. Some patients may struggle to maintain independency following a "minor stroke" [55]. As the stroke patient gains experience and insight in their own outcomes the OT has a part in the rehabilitation process with the purposeful use of activities taking place in the context and environment of relevance to the patient [54].

Fatigue is a factor and should be addressed in order for the patient to manage their time and energy to allow for optimal mastering of their life. Patients with fatigue should followed up, either in the community or as outpatients. Interventions often include help with balancing their energy in daily activities, day planning including rest, and in some cases memory aids.

5.6.2.2 Patients with Moderate to Severe Outcomes

The OT's main objective in the early phase will be to stimulate and guide the patient in simple grooming activities, for example, washing upper body, put on lotion and/or deodorant, brushing the teeth in order to stimulate the level of consciousness, sensibility, perception, and cognition. For patients with severe brain injury it may be beneficial to help them gain increased understanding for the activities by using different stimuli like letting the patient feel the material of the cloth, smell the soap, and so forth. There is evidence that occupational therapy focused on improving personal activities of daily living after stroke can improve performance and reduce risk of deterioration in these abilities [56]. Focused OT should therefore be available to everyone who has had a stroke regardless of the severity of outcomes. The therapy continues with training of motor skills and mobilization to the bedside, practice of balance sitting and standing, and then walking, often in cooperation with the physical therapist and while performing an activity. As motor skills improve the activities and the environment can be graded to increase the challenge for the patient, either within the same activity or with a more demanding activity. Task specific training can be effective to improve upper limb function [57, 58]. Task related training must be based on meaningful activities. For instance, training of the hand with focus on useful grips and natural patterns of movement can be done through gripping a glass, holding it and lifting it up to the mouth. Preferable activities and tasks should be derived from the patient's interests and resources and provide an experience of mastery. Training of cognitive skills must have elements and relevance to daily activities, thus training by the use of known activities should be the focus of occupational therapy [57].

Mr. J—A Neurogeriatrics Case

Mr. J has suffered a stroke and after being assessed in the acute ward he is now in a rehabilitation unit. He has been diagnosed with aphasia by the speech therapist and has some problems understanding instructions and expressing himself. Although he has minor physical outcomes, he has a challenge performing daily activities due to apraxia as reported by the OT. The rehabilitation goals set by himself and aided by the multidisciplinary team are to improve his ability to communicate and be independent in ADL, more specifically eating meals requiring utensils. During lunch he is observed sitting in front of his plate without making an effort to pick up the utensils. Mr. J shows no initiative to act on verbal instructions. The OT then takes his right hand and supports his elbow, moving the right arm and guiding him to grip the knife and moving it towards the butter. He then continues the action and spreads the butter with minor physical guidance from the OT. The OT continues to use this approach of physical guiding the next few days until it is sufficient to push the hand or point towards the knife before the patient grips the knife and starts and using it appropriately. After a couple of weeks the need for physical prompting is gradually decreased and Mr. J becomes more independent in performing various activities requiring tools.

5.6.2.3 Key Elements in Therapeutic Use of Activity in Stroke Rehabilitation

- Avoid unnecessary disturbances
- Tidy up the surroundings and remove unnecessary items and stimuli
- If two people need to be present, define who is "in charge" of the situation
- Grading of help according to the patients' ability
- Give the patient enough time to try to manage a task independently before offering assistance

In Table 5.6 we provide an example of grading of an activity based on the patient's level of performance.

Table 5.6 Example of grading of activities according to the patient's level of performance

• Washing laying/sitting in bed, some activity from patient
• Washing lower body in bed, washing and dressing upper body sitting on bedside/in a wheelchair in the bathroom
• Washing and dressing in the bathroom, help from two lower body
• Washing and dressing in the bathroom, adaptions and help from one person
• Washing and dressing in the bathroom, adaptions and supervision
• Independent, perhaps with some minor adaptions

5.6.3 Special Considerations

Emotional symptoms post-stroke are often neglected and should be addressed as it may affect the rehabilitation process. According to Hildebrand as many as 50% may experience a stroke related psychological or emotional disorder. These symptoms are mainly apathy, reduced motivation, anxiety, fatigue, and sleep disorders similar to symptoms for clinical depression. Complications may arise and must be addressed accordingly. *Edema* may be minimized by elevation of the arm above the heart and/or the use of compression gloves. The use of a sling during mobilization may be considered to avoid *subluxation of the shoulder* when the patient has a paralysis in the upper extremity. *Decubitus* may be prevented by the use of a dynamic air mattress and/or frequent changes of position [59]. Some patients experience reduced orientation and memory. This should be compensated by the use of regular information about time and place. The use of calendars and time tables may give the patient the opportunity to maintain routines and predictability. As well as being a tool to improve orientation it may also give them an increased sense of control.

5.6.3.1 Planning Discharge from Rehabilitation to Home

Towards the end of the rehabilitation process an observation of activity performance may be conducted to evaluate the degree of changes in the quality of performance for the patient. This can be useful to assess the improvement of motor, process, and communication skills and to what extent the patients have reached their goals. This can also identify what amendments need to be done in the home in order for the patient to perform activities independently. At this stage the OT must start the process of obtaining the necessary aids (wheelchair/walker, commode, elevated toilet, etc.). Although the patient is ready to return to their home there will be a need of follow-up and perhaps further rehabilitation in the community. The OT in the community must also be involved if there is a need for home adaptations. In activities associated with I-ADL (communication, banking, shopping, etc.) there is an increased use of technology, also among the older population. However, there is a wide variance of how well the elders use and manage technology in their daily life.

Key Messages

1. Occupational therapy has a unique role in the rehabilitation of elderly patients: promoting their autonomy in activities that are significant for them, even during an acute illness, is useful in improving outcomes and also overall quality of life. Caregivers, with their unique cultural and social background, should always be considered in the rehabilitation process.
2. The occupational therapist, like every other member of the team, should gain specific skills in geriatrics to manage effectively the elderly patients. A specific knowledge of the most common geriatric syndromes is required.

3. To effectively assess and engage patients in the occupational therapy process is crucial to refer to models and assessments of the profession. There are several tools to identify client-centered goals and to recognize factors that could potentially improve the outcomes.

4. Neurodegenerative syndromes should always be considered, as other factors, given their influence on the rehabilitation process. Especially in patients with dementia or Parkinson is crucial to think in a client-centered way determining specific goals that could make the difference in the daily routine of care and in terms of quality of life.

5. Restoring the independence after an orthopedic or neurological condition could be challenging. Assessing the skills that affect the occupational performance of the clients is the first and crucial step before determining client-centered goals. In the rehabilitation process is crucial to grade timing and difficulty of the activities and occupations in which patient is engaged to reach personal goals. Even factors related to setting are important to promote independence and stimulate patients.

References

1. Bachmann S, Finger C, Huss A, Egger M, Stuck AE, Clough-Gorr KM. Inpatient rehabilitation specifically designed for geriatric patients: systematic review and meta-analysis of randomised controlled trials. BMJ. 2010;340:c1718.
2. Goodwin VA, Allan LM. 'Mrs smith has no rehab potential': does rehabilitation have a role in the management of people with dementia? Oxford: Oxford University Press; 2018.
3. Clegg A, Young J, Iliffe S, Rikkert MO, Rockwood K. Frailty in elderly people. Lancet. 2013;381(9868):752–62.
4. Yarnall AJ, Sayer AA, Clegg A, Rockwood K, Parker S, Hindle JV. New horizons in multimorbidity in older adults. Age Ageing. 2017;46(6):882–8.
5. Smit EB, Bouwstra H, Hertogh CM, Wattel EM, van der Wouden JC. Goal-setting in geriatric rehabilitation: a systematic review and meta-analysis. Clin Rehabil. 2019;33(3):395–407.
6. Resnick B, Beaupre L, McGilton KS, Galik E, Liu W, Neuman MD, et al. Rehabilitation interventions for older individuals with cognitive impairment post-hip fracture: a systematic review. J Am Med Dir Assoc. 2016;17(3):200–5.
7. Bellelli G, Morandi A, Gentile S, Trabucchi M. Rehabilitation of elderly adults with severe cognitive impairment: it is time for evidence. J Am Geriatr Soc. 2012;60(5):998–9.
8. Achterberg WP, Cameron ID, Bauer JM, Schols JM. Geriatric rehabilitation—state of the art and future priorities. J Am Med Dir Assoc. 2019;20(4):396–8.
9. Morandi A, Bellelli G, Vasilevskis EE, Turco R, Guerini F, Torpilliesi T, et al. Predictors of rehospitalization among elderly patients admitted to a rehabilitation hospital: the role of polypharmacy, functional status, and length of stay. J Am Med Dir Assoc. 2013;14(10):761–7.
10. Pozzi C, Lucchi E, Lanzoni A, Gentile S, Trabucchi M, Bellelli G, et al. Preliminary evidence of a positive effect of occupational therapy in patients with delirium superimposed on dementia. J Am Med Dir Assoc. 2017;18(12):1091–2.
11. McCloskey R. Functional and self-efficacy changes of patients admitted to a geriatric rehabilitation unit. J Adv Nurs. 2004;46(2):186–93.
12. Coulter A. Paternalism or partnership? Patients have grown up—and there's no going back. BMJ. 1999;319(7212):719–20.
13. Papageorgiou N, Marquis R, Dare J, Batten R. Occupational therapy and occupational participation in community dwelling older adults: a review of the evidence. Phys Occup Ther Geriatr. 2016;34(1):21–42.

14. Law M, Baptiste S, McColl M, Opzoomer A, Polatajko H, Pollock N. The Canadian occupational performance measure: an outcome measure for occupational therapy. Can J Occup Ther. 1990;57(2):82–7.
15. Everink IH, van Haastregt JC, Maessen JM, Schols JM, Kempen GI. Process evaluation of an integrated care pathway in geriatric rehabilitation for people with complex health problems. BMC Health Serv Res. 2017;17(1):34.
16. Josephsson S, Bäckman L, Borell L, Bernspång B, Nygård L, Rönnberg L. Supporting everyday activities in dementia: an intervention study. Int J Geriatr Psychiatry. 1993;8(5):395–400.
17. Smallfield S, Heckenlaible C. Effectiveness of occupational therapy interventions to enhance occupational performance for adults with Alzheimer's disease and related major neurocognitive disorders: a systematic review. Am J Occup Ther. 2017;71(5):7105180010p1–9.
18. de Werd MM, Boelen D, Rikkert MGO, Kessels RP. Errorless learning of everyday tasks in people with dementia. Clin Interv Aging. 2013;8:1177.
19. Buettner L, Kolanowski A. Prescribing activities that engage passive residents: an innovative method. J Gerontol Nurs. 2008;34(1):13–8.
20. National Collaborating Centre for Mental Health. Dementia: a NICE-SCIE guideline on supporting people with dementia and their carers in health and social care. Leicester: British Psychological Society; 2007.
21. Gitlin LN, Winter L, Burke J, Chernett N, Dennis MP, Hauck WW. Tailored activities to manage neuropsychiatric behaviors in persons with dementia and reduce caregiver burden: a randomized pilot study. Am J Geriatr Psychiatry. 2008;16(3):229–39.
22. Samii A, Nutt JG, Ransom BR. Parkinson's disease. Lancet. 2004;363(9423):1783–93.
23. Foster ER, Bedekar M, Tickle-Degnen L. Systematic review of the effectiveness of occupational therapy–related interventions for people with Parkinson's disease. Am J Occup Ther. 2014;68(1):39–49.
24. Sturkenboom IH, Graff MJ, Borm GF, Adang EM, Nijhuis-van der Sanden MW, Bloem BR, et al. Effectiveness of occupational therapy in Parkinson's disease: study protocol for a randomized controlled trial. Trials. 2013;14(1):34.
25. Abbruzzese G, Marchese R, Avanzino L, Pelosin E. Rehabilitation for Parkinson's disease: current outlook and future challenges. Parkinsonism Relat Disord. 2016;22:S60–S4.
26. Foster ER, Hershey T. Everyday executive function is associated with activity participation in Parkinson disease without dementia. OTJR. 2011;31(1_suppl):S16–22.
27. Sturkenboom I, Thijssen M, Gons-van Elsacker J, Maasdam A, Schulten M, Vijver-Visser D, et al. Guidelines for occupational therapy in Parkinson's disease rehabilitation. Nijmegen/Miami, FL: ParkinsonNet/NPF Heruntergeladen von; 2011;3:2016. http://www.parkinsonnet/info/media/14820461/ot_guidelines_final-npf__3_.pdf.
28. Association AP. Diagnostic and statistical manual of mental disorders (DSM-5®). Washington, DC: American Psychiatric Publishing; 2013.
29. Inouye SK, Bogardus ST Jr, Charpentier PA, Leo-Summers L, Acampora D, Holford TR, et al. A multicomponent intervention to prevent delirium in hospitalized older patients. N Engl J Med. 1999;340(9):669–76.
30. Álvarez EA, Garrido MA, Tobar EA, Prieto SA, Vergara SO, Briceño CD, et al. Occupational therapy for delirium management in elderly patients without mechanical ventilation in an intensive care unit: a pilot randomized clinical trial. J Crit Care. 2017;37:85–90.
31. Inouye SK, Foreman MD, Mion LC, Katz KH, Cooney LM Jr. Nurses' recognition of delirium and its symptoms: comparison of nurse and researcher ratings. Arch Intern Med. 2001;161(20):2467–73.
32. Spronk PE, Riekerk B, Hofhuis J, Rommes JH. Occurrence of delirium is severely underestimated in the ICU during daily care. Intensive Care Med. 2009;35(7):1276–80.
33. Morandi A, McCurley J, Vasilevskis EE, Fick DM, Bellelli G, Lee P, et al. Tools to detect delirium superimposed on dementia: a systematic review. J Am Geriatr Soc. 2012;60(11):2005–13.
34. Bellelli G, Morandi A, Davis DH, Mazzola P, Turco R, Gentile S, et al. Validation of the 4AT, a new instrument for rapid delirium screening: a study in 234 hospitalised older people. Age Ageing. 2014;43(4):496–502.

35. Inouye SK, van Dyck CH, Alessi CA, Balkin S, Siegal AP, Horwitz RI. Clarifying confusion: the confusion assessment method: a new method for detection of delirium. Ann Intern Med. 1990;113(12):941–8.
36. Ely EW, Truman B, Shintani A, Thomason JW, Wheeler AP, Gordon S, et al. Monitoring sedation status over time in ICU patients: reliability and validity of the Richmond Agitation-Sedation Scale (RASS). JAMA. 2003;289(22):2983–91.
37. Fisher A. Occupational therapy intervention process model. Fort Collins, CO: Three Star Press, Inc; 2009.
38. Scottish Intercollegiate Guidelines Network (SIGN).SIGN157 Risk reduction andmanagement of delirium. Edinburgh: SIGN; 2019. (SIGN publication no. 157). [cited 28 11 2019]. Available from URL: http://www.sign.ac.uk.
39. Bertram M, Norman R, Kemp L, Vos T. Review of the long-term disability associated with hip fractures. Inj Prev. 2011;17(6):365–70.
40. Ranhoff AH, Holvik K, Martinsen MI, Domaas K, Solheim LF. Older hip fracture patients: three groups with different needs. BMC Geriatr. 2010;10(1):65.
41. (NICE) TNIfHaCE. Hip fracture: management, C. G. (CG124). 2017. Available from: https://www.nice.org.uk/guidance/cg124. Accessed 2 Aug 2019.
42. Therapy CoO. Occupational therapy in prevention and management of fall in adults. www.rcot.co.uk: UK.
43. Tarazona Santabalbina FJ, Belenguer-Varea Á, Rovina E, Cuesta-Peredo D. Orthogeriatric care: improving patient outcomes. Clin Interv Aging. 2016;11:843–56.
44. Juliebø V, Bjøro K, Krogseth M. Risk factors for preoperative and postoperative delirium in elderly patients with hip fracture. Am Geriatr Soc. 2009;57:1354–62.
45. CG124 N. Hip fracture: management. In: (CG124) CG, editor. https://www.nice.org.uk/guidance/cg124. The National Institute for Health Care Excellence; 2017.
46. Crennan MM. Occupatioanl therapy discharge assessment of elderly patients from acute care hospitals. Phys Occup Ther Geriatr. 2010;28(1):33–43.
47. Edwards M, Baptiste S, Stratford PW, Law M. Recovery after hip fracture: what can we learn from Canadian occupational performance measure. Am J Occup Ther. 2007;61:335–44.
48. Lenze EJ, Munin MC, Dew MA, Rogers JC, Seligman K, Mulsant BH, et al. Adverse effects of depression and cognitive impairment on rehabilitation participation and recovery from hip fracture. Int J Geriatr Psychiatry. 2004;19(5):472–8.
49. Lenze E, Munin MV, Dew MA, Rogers JC, Seligmann K, Musant BH, Reynolds CF 3rd. Adverse effects of depression and cognitive impairment on rehabilitation, participation and recovery from hip fracture. Int J Geriatr Psychiatry. 2004;19(5):472–8.
50. Grue EV, Kirkvold M, Ranhoff AH. Prevalence of vision, hearing and combined vision and hearing impairments with hip fractures. J Clin Nurs. 2009;18(21):3037–49.
51. Inouyw S, Westendorp RG, Saczynsi JS. Delirium in elderly people. Lancet. 2014;383: 911–22.
52. Health TNDo. Norwegian guidelines on management and rehabilitation of stroke. 2010. Available from: http://www.helsebiblioteket.no/Retningslinjer/Hjerneslag/Forord-og-innledning.
53. Fure B, Engebretsen E, Thommessen B, Øksengård A, Brækhus A. Clinical neurological examination of the geriatric patient. Tidsskr Nor Laegeforen. 2011;131(11):1080–3.
54. Wolf TJ, Baum C, Connor LT. Changing face of stroke: implications for occupational therapy practice. Am J Occup Ther. 2009;63(5):621.
55. Graven C, Sansonetti D, Moloczij N, Cadilhac D, Joubert L. Stroke survivor and carer perspectives of the concept of recovery: a qualitative study. Disabil Rehabil. 2013;35(7):578–85.
56. Legg L, Drummond A, Leonardi-Bee J, Gladman J, Corr S, Donkervoort M, et al. Occupational therapy for patients with problems in personal activities of daily living after stroke: systematic review of randomised trials. BMJ. 2007;335(7626):922.

57. Quinn TJ, Paolucci S, Sunnerhagen KS, Sivenius J, Walker MF, Toni D, et al. Evidence-based stroke rehabilitation: an expanded guidance document from the European Stroke Organisation (ESO) guidelines for management of ischaemic stroke and transient ischaemic attack 2008. J Rehabil Med. 2009;41(2):99–111.
58. Wattchow KA, McDonnell MN, Hillier SL. Rehabilitation interventions for upper limb function in the first four weeks following stroke: a systematic review and meta-analysis of the evidence. Arch Phys Med Rehabil. 2018;99(2):367–82.
59. Berlowitz D, Schmader KE. Clinical staging and management of pressure-induced skin and soft tissue injury. In: UpToDate. Waltham, MA. Accessed 14 Dec 2018.

Occupational Therapy in Nursing Home

Barbara Manni, Laura Gitlin, Glenda Garzetta,
Lesley Collier, and Andrea Fabbo

6.1 Introduction

Greater longevity has increased the demand for chronic care in a frail population of older people. Maintaining functionality is important not only for self-independence but also for prevention of caregiver burden. Loss of independence or excessive caregiver burden is the cause of institutionalization, mainly in case of people of dementia and neuropsychiatric symptoms (NPS). Lower quality of life (QOL) of elderly people in nursing homes (NH) was linked to their dissatisfaction with the capacity to make decisions, a monotonous life, loss of physical and mental autonomy, and nutritional deviations [1, 2]. Many care homes provide excellent care but the depersonalizing environment, negative staff attitudes, and lack of meaningful occupation can have a detrimental impact on resident's physical and mental well-being.

B. Manni (⊠) · G. Garzetta · A. Fabbo
Primary Care Department, Cognitive Disorders and Dementia Unit, Health Authority
and Services of Modena, AUSL, Modena, Italy
e-mail: ba.manni@ausl.mo.it

L. Gitlin
College of Nursing and Health Professions, Drexel University, Philadelphia, PA, USA
e-mail: lgitlin1@jhu.edu

L. Collier
College of Health and Life Sciences, Brunel University, London, UK
e-mail: lesley.collier@brunel.ac.uk

© Springer Nature Switzerland AG 2020
C. Pozzi et al. (eds.), *Occupational Therapy for Older People*,
https://doi.org/10.1007/978-3-030-35731-3_6

6.2   Importance of Activities and Social Engagement and the Role of the Occupational Therapist for Older People with Dementia in Nursing Homes

Quality of life in nursing homes (NH) is strictly related to personal, organizational, activity-related, and social factors. In a Belgian NH study, cognitively healthy residents declared satisfaction in quality of life relating to subjective self-perception of general health, mood, social engagement (considered as relationship with peer and staff), engagement in routine activities, and access to meaningful activities [3]. "Meaningful occupation" has been defined as having a wide range of activities that are meaningful for a person. An activity is meaningful if this is significant to, or valued by, the person and provides enjoyment, a sense of purpose, belonging, or achievement.

The ability to participate in valued activities, whether for work, leisure, or family, is an important aspect of personal identity. In dementia, progressive memory loss means that abilities developed over a lifetime begin to lose as well, contributing to the loss of self and identity. When admitted in NH people with dementia experiment social withdrawal, reduced engagement in active and passive activities that result in low quality of life perception [1]. Occupational therapist in NH also plays an important role against residents' loneliness and identity loss in people with dementia because it promotes activity engagement interventions and other non-pharmacological multicomponent interventions improving quality of life, functioning (activities of daily life, ADL), and enhances significant personal activities, hobbies, and values resulting in reduction of medication and restraints [2, 4, 5]. Occupational therapist also considers a global life approach to residents with dementia according to the "Person Centered Care" approach [6] which asks for a cultural change in attitudes of all staff in nursing homes. Person Centered Care means considering the person before considering the illness. Person-centered care (PCC) has emerged as an alternative way of caring for someone with dementia, and shifts the attention from the behavior to what may be causing or contributing to the behavior. PCC approach prevents and improves challenging behaviors, agitation, depression, and quality of life in people with dementia independently of stage and setting [7, 8] and demonstrates a good cost-effectiveness [9].

The cultural change movement aims to deconstruct the medical model for nursing homes replacing it with a more homelike atmosphere in which nursing home operations are centered around the needs and desires of individual residents. Its main principles are to make resident choices and preferences guide all aspects of daily life; to ensure that residents, staff members, families, and the broader community develop close bonds; to make the nursing home environment more like the homes residents used to live in as opposed to a hospital; and to continually improve the quality of care. "Culture change" is often used synonymously with "person-centered care" (PCC), as it will be here [10]. A PCC approach is important also in activities proposed to residents. Implementing tailored meaningful activities for residents of care homes showed more health, well-being (depression reduction, less use of catheters, minor risk of pressure ulcers, and use of physical restraints) [11], and quality of life [9, 12].

Occupational therapist plays an important role in implementing educational strategies that include learning and skill development of internal staff in NH. PCC training can have positive influence on stress and burn out staff reduction and job satisfaction [8].

6.3 Meaningful Activity Refers to a Range of Activities (Physical, Social, Cognitive, Leisure Activities) Tailored to a Person's Needs and Preferences

In NH there are complex and multilevel barriers to engaging in activities. To deliver effective and person centered activity programs in NH it is necessary to consider individual needs and preferences and organizational and environmental barriers while empowering and educating staff. When people with dementia are admitted to a care home social engaging gets complicated. Professionals are busy and involved in care; recreational therapists have less time to spend in individual care activities; people with dementia often present severe cognitive impairment and it is difficult for professionals to know each person's biography, hobbies, or interest. Engaging in activities in NH, on the other side, is not so easy in particular for people living with cognitive impairment. There are a lot of barriers such as difficulties in engaging, because of apathy or excess in agitation, discouraging or too much difficult activities in respect of cognitive level, difficulties in satisfying every personal areas of interest or the correct daily moment to practice it. Agitated or passive older with dementia can be difficult to involve in activities which means they are at risk for isolation, use of restraints, cognitive and functional decline and staff care's frustration. An advanced stage of dementia reflects loss of identity and communication problems that interfere with the capacity of professionals to satisfy personal needs. Activities that are meaningful for people with dementia are similar to those for people without dementia and include a wide variety of leisure and recreational activities, household chores, social involvement, and work related activities. Meaningful activities create a feeling of pleasure and enjoyment and a sense of connection and belonging and promoting a sense of autonomy and personal identity.

Moyra Jones in her "Gentle Care" theory [13] introduces the concept of indoors and outdoors environments and the importance of daily activities plans. We know that people living with Alzheimer disease experience a progressively lowered stress threshold [14], which means reduced ability to cope with stress. The environment can be a partner or an enemy in particular in NH. Occupational therapists can help to suggest environmental changes in order to help cognitive disability. Therapist considers every enviromental element; such as how the furniture has placed or sensory input (noises, lights, temperature, colors), that can be confortable or unconfortable for people with dementia related to preferences, needs and cognitive level. Moreover, according to the PCC model it is important to plan activities considering cognitive level, biography and personal preferences, and relaxing time. It is important to find an activity able to motivate and involve client, not discourage or bore. Occupational therapist's skill takes care to avoid excess or lack of stimuli that can encourage agitation or boredom and considers personhood and personality of the client.

His multilevel role helps to plan environmental changes, to consider barriers and facilitators to resident's participation in activities, and to train staff in educational strategies to avoid resident distress [15].

A person-centered treatment by occupational therapist in a community-dwelling people affected by dementia has demonstrated positive effects. For example in the COTiD method (community based occupational therapy for patients with mild–moderate dementia) occupational therapist plays an important role in examining patient and caregiver's needs and identifying cognitive and behavioral interventions in people with dementia to compensate for cognitive decline and to support pleasure and social engagement [16, 17]. A pilot experience of the method in residential setting demonstrated benefits for people with moderate and severe dementia and challenging behavior. The problem solving approach of the occupational therapist considers people with dementia's habits and meaningful activities and both formal (care assistant) and informal caregiver's point of view. The therapist who uses the COTiD method, ends the home visit drafting a personal daily care program that includes people with dementia in a daily routine [18].

6.3.1   Which Kind of Activities Are Recommended Regarding Different Stage of Dementia?

Little is currently known about what specific characteristics of an activity can enhance an individual's ability to be meaningfully engaged. A recent study [19] analyzed a group of people with dementia in different stages of disease with behavioral problems such as boredom, sadness, anxiety, agitation, restlessness, or difficulty in focusing on task and caregivers. This study considers seven different kind of activities proposed by occupational therapist to people with dementia in different levels of cognitive performance and functioning disabilities. The activities considered were: arts and crafts (e.g., refinishing wood bench and coloring pictures), physical exercise (e.g., pedal pusher exerciser and walking), cognitive (e.g., concentration card game and puzzles), music and entertainment (e.g., watching vintage movies and listening to music), manipulation/sensory/sorting (e.g., activity pillow and sorting jewelry), family/social/reminiscence (e.g., family photo album, reminiscing, and visiting family), and domestic/homemaking (e.g., folding laundry and preparing snacks).

Three groups responded in different ways in order to engaging time, pleasure, necessity of cues or redirection of task or initiating help. In Fig. 6.1, we described which stage of cognitive disease better responded to the activity proposed:

Persons with severe cognitive impairment may benefit from sensory-type activities such as bouncing a balloon, listening to music, or watching videos of animals. Persons with moderate cognitive impairment may benefit from procedural activities or activities using repetitive actions such as washing dishes, sorting beads or cards; whereas persons with mild dementia may benefit from goal-directed activities such as arts and crafts, preparing simple meals, painting, or puzzles. Persons with mild dementia were most often prescribed complex activities like art and craft and cognitive tasks that require sequencing and problem solving skills. The purpose of activity is to engage the person and provide a pleasant experience to promote a sense of self, connectedness, belonging, and identity with disease progression [19].

Type of activity	Mild dementia	Moderate dementia	Severe dementia
Arts and craft	🟩	🟨	🟥
Exercise/physical	🟥	🟨	🟩
Cognitive	🟩	🟨	🟥
Music/Entertainment	🟥	🟩	🟨
Manipulation/sensory /sorting	🟨	🟥	🟩
Family/social	🟩	🟨	🟥
Domestic/ homemaking	🟥	🟩	🟨

Fig. 6.1 Different response in different tasks regarding different stage of dementia. Red color means most difficulties in involving in activity or less prescribed, yellow color means moderate engagement in activity, green color means most prescribed and pleasure engagement in activity

6.4   Role of Occupational Therapy in Managing Challenging Behavior of People with Dementia in Nursing Home

Engaging in activity becomes difficult as cognitive decline gets worse in people with dementia and it is necessary to personalize intervention. In people with challenging behavior, this concept is most important. Behavioral and psychological symptoms of dementia (BPSD) are unavoidable and logic reactions to unmet needs, mismatches between a person's capabilities and caregiver, or environmental expectation. They result from internal (neurodegenerative processes, premorbid personality, etc.) and external factors. External factors depend on the environmental (setting, overcrowding, noises, lights, etc.) and the caregiver relationship. Caregiver sometimes cannot understand the link between dementia and BPSD and they believe they have this behavior "on purpose," or they have an ineffective communication style or unrealistic expectation. These feelings reflect a wrong communication with people with dementia who feel inadequacy, sadness, or angry against caregiver. Moreover, some families can experience the NH placement of their loved ones with a sense of guilt that reflects in unrealistic expectations for care and assistance.

In nursing home BPSD (in particular agitation, anxiety, and aggression), language impairments, taking psychotropic drugs, and lower levels of self-care are associated with reduced wellbeing.

Behavioral symptoms occur across disease etiologies and stages. Symptoms result in negative sequela including increased healthcare costs, reduced quality of life and functional dependence, rapid disease progression and more time spent caregiving, nursing home placement, and caregiver distress [20]. People with dementia and BPSD are clients most associated with difficulties to manage, one of the most important factors that influence burnout in NH staff [21]. The Food and Drug Administration has not approved any pharmacological treatments for these patients in the recent years. Off-label antipsychotic medications prescribed have risks, including stroke and mortality, that often outweigh their modest benefits.

One promising non-pharmacologic approach is the use of activities that capitalize on preserved capabilities and life-long social roles and interests. Evidence suggests that persons with dementia can effectively engage in activities graded to their abilities resulting in reduced NPS [5] and use of antipsychotic drugs in NH [22].

Psychosocial interventions (reminiscence, personalized music, personalized activities with or without social interaction, validation therapy, PCC training) are found to improve mood, agitation, apathy, increase pleasure and interest independently from social interaction in people with dementia in any stage [23, 24]. In this frail population in particular if BPSD are diagnosed, it is most important to implement a Person Centered Care approach and to propose person centered activities. Like this and thanks to involvement of NH staff it is possible to aim an improvement in quality of life in residents [25]. In this case, occupational therapist plays an important role; he is an expert in understanding the explicit relationship between person, environment, and occupation required for a successful task performance.

Other positive results are described by Collier in using of Snoezelen (multisensory behavior therapy) in management of BPSD in moderate–severe stages; in particular in reducing agitation, anxiety, and apathy and increasing in activities of daily living in clinical setting and in homecare [26, 27]. In the home setting, Tailored Activity Program (TAP) Method by Gitlin et al., they demonstrated positive immediate effects of occupational therapy on NPS, functional dependence and pain in people with dementia, and decrease of caregiver distress [28, 29]. Occupational therapists in this case have a key role in catching residual capabilities, improving executive and physical functioning, and evaluating fall risk and environment (lighting, seating, clutter, noise). After 6 home visits the occupational therapist creates a report and prescribes the most significant, pleasant activities of the resident in a daily plan. Moreover, occupational therapists teach caregivers how to simplify and propose activities, how to change communication, and how to manage situational distress and understand and deal with challenging behavior [28, 29].

Ideally, the non-pharmacological approach to BPSD in clinical setting occurs in a multidisciplinary team. It expresses a collaborative care model in which trigger figures are involved, such as trained nurses, recreational therapists, occupational therapists, and geriatrician. At the beginning, occupational therapist interviews families about patient's habits and interests, explores environmental barriers, and analyzes patient's capabilities and risk of falls. In a second time, the therapist prescribes tailored activities conveying patient deficits and interests. The last phase occupational therapists engage nurses and recreational therapists to observe and try to practice with the specific activity. The occupational therapist moreover encourages continued activity use and helps generalizing strategy use to other difficult situations to cope with challenging behavior. The same training has to be done to familiars before discharge. This study observed a good engagement with pleasure and positive behavioral outcomes, less anxiety, restlessness, and anger of patient during treatment [30].

The method could be copied in NH with specific training programs addressed to NH staff, but at the moment more studies are needed to verify applicability of TAP model in NH setting. Even in this case, in a long care setting it is necessary to have a collaborative multidisciplinary team to implement an approach of a non-pharmacological treatment of NPS. DICE (Describe, Investigate, Create, and Evaluate) approach is a person and caregiver centered method for management of challenging behavior in people with dementia in home care setting [31]. This integrated model described in Fig. 6.2 was outlined by a team including a geriatrician, psychiatry, psychologist, expert in pharmacy, and a nurse. It is a guide for occupational therapists and it focuses on people with dementia, the caregiver, and the environment.

Step 1 **DESCRIBE**	The team analyzes the characterization of the NPS and the context in which it occurs, the antecedents and consequences. The Occupational Therapist analysis includes a review of patient abilities, environmental setting and formal/informal communications and interactions.
Step 2 **INVESTIGATE**	The team detect underlying and modifiable causes such as illness or pain, medication side effects, prior psychiatric comorbidity, limitations in functioning, poor sleep hygiene, sensory deficits, boredom, feeling of inadequacy. Occupational therapists should assess cognitive, motor and functional abilities, risk of falls and examine patient's routines, preferences, occupation, hobbies, cultural and religious contest. Moreover they have to analyze the environment.
Step 3 **CREATE**	A treatment plan should be created involving the professional team, the caregiver and person with dementia, if possible. The physician responds to physical problems, pain management and reviews the medication scheme. Aids should also use to reduce sensory impairments. Problem solving strategies are directed to eliminating specific NPS (e.g. aggression at the bath) while a-specific and global interventions arranged by occupational therapist are effective to prevent NPS onset,it contains of caregiver education, enhancing effective communication, involving the patient in meaningful activities and to simplify tasks and establish routines.
Step 4 **EVALUATE**	It's important to evaluate the positive or negative effects and the efficacy of treatment. The Occupational therapist has the role to implement strategies, analyze which and why strategies worked or not worked and to follow up behavior reporting to team and physician every changes.

Fig. 6.2 DICE model as a multidisciplinary and collaborative care model for challenging behavior in residents with dementia

BPSD management in people with dementia in NH has to be multilevel and multiprofessional management. Only in a multidisciplinary approach we can consider every aspect of a multidimensional problem as in case of challenging behavior.

Occupational meaningful engagement should be a primary aim in a resident daily plan in NH even in case of cognitive impairment. An activity can be designed for a person at any level of impairment as long as they are responsive to their environment. Progressively cognitive impairment asks for activities to become simple, divided into one or two step type with eventual use of auditive and tactile cues to support initiating and sequencing. Meaningful activities become most important in case of challenging behavior because they can promote pleasure and reduce boredom or agitation. Involvement of occupational therapist in every NH's organization should be promoted to upgrade quality of life of residents.

6.5 Focus on Dementia and BPSD: The Tailor Activity Program (T.A.P.)

As this case snapshot illustrates, behavioral and psychological symptoms (BPSD) such as irritability, wandering, rejection of care among others, are common core clinical features of dementia. BPSD are practically universal, occur regardless of etiology and throughout the disease trajectory, and can be disturbing to persons themselves and their care partners. For persons living with dementia, untreated BPSD have been associated with more rapid disease progression, greater morbidity and mortality, higher rates of hospital and health care utilization, and relocation to residential care [32–34]. For family caregivers, BPSD have been associated with increased caregiver burden [35], upset, depression and stress, and decreased quality of life. By the moderate disease stage, some studies have shown that caregivers may be managing anywhere from six to 12 different behavioral manifestations. The management of four or more behavioral symptoms at any one time reflects a tipping point in which caregivers begin to report clinical depression and burden [36, 37].

6.5.1 Why Do Behavioral and Psychological Symptoms in Dementia Occur?

It is unclear why BPSD occur with dementia. A conceptual model developed by a working group sponsored by the National Institutes of Health in the USA suggests that with neurodegeneration, disruptions in brain circuitry, and decrements in information processing and executive function, persons with dementia become increasingly vulnerable to potentially modifiable internal and external factors that may contribute to BPSD. These factors include those related to the person living with dementia, the caregiver, and/or the living environment [38].

Person-based factors might include for example untreated pain or infection, side effects of medications, boredom, feelings of insecurity, loss of control and/or a sense of purpose, fatigue, or having unmet needs of basic daily living such as hunger, thirst, being too hot or cold. Furthermore, having pain, underlying infections, or blood disorders can also contribute to BPSD. A study of 256 community-dwelling people with dementia found that 36% of those in an intervention group had an undetected illness associated with agitation, repeated questioning, crying out, delusions, and/or hallucinations [39, 40].

Caregiver factors that may impact BPSD include but are not limited to the use of overly complex communications, poor health, or being highly stressed/overwhelmed. Factors related to physical environments include ambient noise, light levels, temperature conditions, over or under-stimulation, insufficient lighting, and/or clutter.

Of importance is that these person, caregiver and environmental-based factors are modifiable, suggesting that strategies that address these potential contributors may reduce, eliminate, or manage targeted behaviors. Given the complexity of the etiology for any one behavior (e.g., it may be due to an underlying infection plus a cluttered environment and overwhelmed caregiver), a simple "magic bullet" solution such as a medication for all BPSD is highly unlikely. Although there are no officially approved medications to treat BPSD, a common clinical practice in most countries and settings is the use of psychiatric medications (e.g., antipsychotics, anticonvulsants). This is the case even though antipsychotic medications show very modest efficacy in improving BPSD and have significant risks including side effects and mortality which has resulted in an FDA black box warning in the USA for using these medications for this purpose [41, 42]. Additionally, medications like anticonvulsants are currently being used as alternatives to antipsychotics although they have similar risks and even less evidence of benefit [43]. In contrast, a plethora of non-pharmacologic strategies have been shown to be efficacious. Their use has been endorsed by many medical associations worldwide as the preferred first-line treatment, except in emergency situations, when behaviors might lead to imminent danger to the person or carer [44]. Nevertheless, few clinicians and families are aware of such approaches, have access to proven programs designed to mitigate BPSD, or understand how to select a non-pharmacologic strategy. In primary care, despite quality measures recommending ascertainment of BPSD and caregiver education in their management, this rarely occurs due to a number of factors including time constraints, practical knowledge, and/or payment structures which limit reimbursement for practitioner time in engaging in education and skills training [45]. Also, as most approaches rely on a systematic approach to identifying specific triggers for a behavior followed by developing a treatment plan involving caregiver education, these approaches can be time-consuming, labor-intensive, costly, and effective for a short time frame despite the long trajectory of family care provision and behavioral management needs. Additionally, most proven approaches have been tested outside of the service context thus necessitating translation into a deliverable and sustained service, leaving most families underserved and health professionals on their own to figure out how to manage behaviors.

6.5.2 What Is the Role of Occupational Therapists?

Occupational therapists have a significant role in dementia care and helping families and formal providers prevent, reduce, and/or manage behavioral symptoms [31]. As occupational therapists are skilled in understanding human behavior within the context of the person's life space, they are uniquely qualified to assess for and modify potential contributors to BPSD. For example, occupational therapists can assess for executive function and instruct caregivers as to how to use a wide range of cueing techniques to help a person living with dementia to initiate, plan, organize, and/or sequence a particular activity. An inability to initiate or carry out an activity can serve as a source of agitation for persons living with dementia. Additionally, therapists can assess the living environment and whether it provides a supportive context for the person with dementia vis-à-vis their particular abilities and disease stage. Therapists can also evaluate the communication and management style of caregivers, provide disease education, and help caregivers modify their style to meet the needs of the person living with dementia. Additionally, therapists can help family members better understand the disease and its implications for everyday living as well as introduce strategies for taking care of themselves.

6.5.3 The Tailored Activity Program

One promising non-pharmacologic approach that has been developed with occupational therapists to address behavioral symptoms is the use of activities that are tailored to the interests and abilities of persons living with dementia. As the heart of occupational therapy is activity use, task analysis, and grading activities to abilities, this particular program highly resonates with the basic scope of practice and skill set of this profession. The program, New Ways for Better Days: Tailoring Activities for Persons with Dementia and their Caregivers (or Tailored Activity Program—TAP for short) draws upon occupational therapy principles including activity analysis and simplification, person-centered care, problem solving, and person–environment fit [46, 47].

TAP has been evaluated in a variety of settings including the home, hospital, adult day services, assisted living, and other residential care contexts. Taken as a whole, studies have shown significant benefit for persons with dementia including reduced agitated and other behavioral symptoms, maintenance of daily function, improved quality of life and engagement; and for caregivers, studies have shown time savings, improved overall well-being and quality of life [29, 48].

In Fig. 6.3 there is a description of the three Phases for the application of the TAP. In Phase I, assessment (up to two sessions), the occupational therapist evaluates the preserved abilities and interests of persons living with dementia, caregiver (formal and/or family) communication styles, coping mechanisms, and readiness to use new strategies, and their availability as well as the setup of the physical environment (level of clutter, lighting, seating, areas where activities may occur). Caregivers receive educational resources including the Caregiver Guide to Dementia: Using

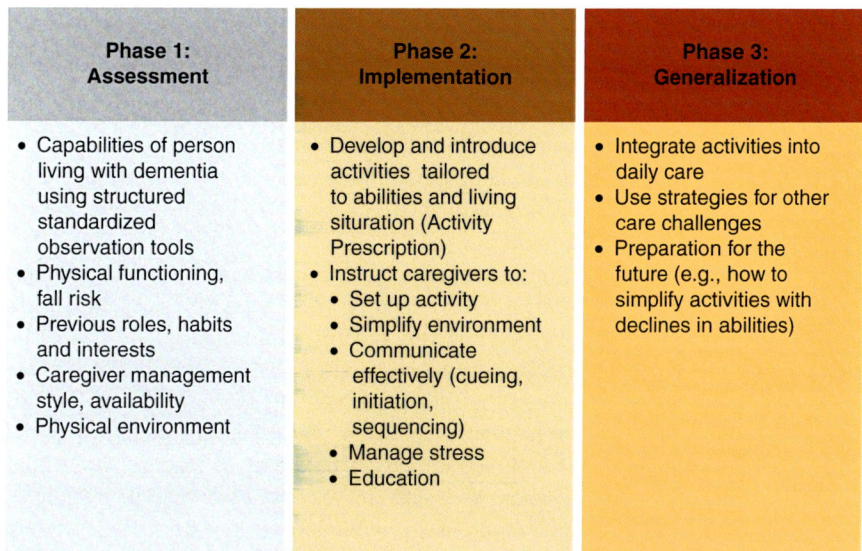

Phase 1: Assessment	Phase 2: Implementation	Phase 3: Generalization

• Capabilities of person living with dementia using structured standardized observation tools
• Physical functioning, fall risk
• Previous roles, habits and interests
• Caregiver management style, availability
• Physical environment
	• Develop and introduce activities tailored to abilities and living situation (Activity Prescription)
	• Instruct caregivers to:
	  • Set up activity
	  • Simplify environment
	  • Communicate effectively (cueing, initiation, sequencing)
	  • Manage stress
	  • Education
		• Integrate activities into daily care
		• Use strategies for other care challenges
		• Preparation for the future (e.g., how to simplify activities with declines in abilities)

Fig. 6.3 Three phases of the application of the Tailored Activity Program (TAP) [46, 47]

Activities and other Strategies to Manage Behavioral Symptoms [49]. This booklet provides tips for addressing behavioral symptoms in the form of helpful checklists and recommendations for taking care of self as a caregiver and medical considerations in the care of persons with dementia (e.g., monitoring hydration, pain, medications). Also, the occupational therapist introduces simple stress reduction techniques (deep breathing) to help caregivers manage situational stress and set a calm tone in the environment prior to their use of activities as a therapeutic tool.

Activities are identified based on the assessment outcomes and are case specific. They may include but are not limited to crafts (painting/coloring, bead work), preparing a simple meal, sorting objects, walking, gardening, placing flowers in a vase, listening to music, viewing a soothing video, or manipulating sensory-type objects for individuals. Activities are graded to the cognitive, functional, social, and interest profiles of persons living with dementia with consideration also given to physical and social environmental factors, such as the location in which an activity should occur (e.g., dining room table, in a well-lit area), caregiver availability, understanding of dementia and time needed to setup or supervise activities, and so forth.

In Phase II, the occupational therapist provides the caregiver (formal or family member) with a written assessment report that summarizes the results of Phase I assessments using lay terms in order to set the ground work for helping caregivers understand the capabilities of the person with dementia or what they can do and cannot do and types of supports needed. The therapist also prepares an "Activity Prescription" for each identified activity. This written document summarizes in lay language the capabilities of the person with dementia (e.g., good coordination and use of arms and hands), the activity (e.g., folding towels), when and where and for how long to conduct the activity (e.g., 20 min twice daily while caregiver prepares lunch and dinner meals), and specific instructions for introducing and using the activity. Specific instructions may include how to set up the activity, modify the environment, and communicate effectively.

Caregivers are further instructed in how to integrate activities into daily routines (time of day, number of times per week, potential length of an activity session). One activity is introduced per session although all three can also be introduced in cases where the number of sessions is truncated or caregiver is of high readiness and able to absorb the information provided.

In Phase III, caregivers learn how to simplify each activity with cognitive declines and how to use strategies (e.g., simplify environment, relax the rules) to address other care challenges (e.g., rejection of care, repetitive questioning).

While caregivers receive all treatment phases, the pace by which TAP progresses depends upon caregiver readiness and the acceptability and use of each activity. Caregivers with a low level of readiness (e.g., poor understanding of dementia, view of behaviors as intentional, depressed, or very overwhelmed) tend to overestimate the abilities of the person for whom they care and may not easily gravitate to the use of activity. In these cases, interventionists provide more education and demonstration of how changing communications or simplifying an activity can yield positive results. Caregivers who are at a high level of readiness tend to have a good understanding of dementia and the abilities of the person they care for and move more quickly through sessions and adapt easily to the structure of the program and activities being offered. An online program has now been developed for this program for a fee and can be accessed at: http://learn.nursing.jhu.edu/face-to-face/institutes/NewWay-TAP/index.html. In Fig. 6.4 we provide testimonials of caregivers involved in the TAP program.

TAP is being deployed in numerous countries including Scotland, Italy, Brazil, Chile, Australia, Hong Kong, Russia, and the USA. Outcomes may vary by country, but the testimonials as shown in Fig. 6.4 are similar. Adaptations to TAP are permissible and often necessary depending upon the setting in which it is embedded and culture and country as outlined in Table 6.1.

Testimonials from TAP Caregivers
"He really enjoyed singing along with Frank Sinatra. He wasn't really enjoying anything else but those girls (OTs) worked hard to help him. They were the best part of the whole time there." (Wife, Hospital Setting)
"It helped the residents get through their time here and it helped me to keep (the patient's) mind occupied and keep them calm. I think it is a wonderful program. (GNA, Hospital setting)
"That (the cooking activity) is still the one thing my dad asks to help with every day. I'm still using the breathing and imagery --- your help has meant such an improvement in our quality of life--- (Daughter, Home Setting)"
"I feel very lucky to have participated in TAP. I think that I learned a lot, and everything has helped me deal with the situation in a much more effective way." (Daughter, Home Setting)

Fig. 6.4 Testimonials from TAP caregivers

Although adaptations such as those identified in Table 6.1 are permissible and reflect the flexibility of the program, there are immutable principles that must be adhered to and these are outlined in Fig. 6.5. These principles make the TAP effective or reflect its "mechanism of action" and assure relevancy and appropriateness of the program per family.

In summary, behavioral and psychological symptoms are a core clinical feature of dementia that may reflect expressions, heightened sensitivity, and vulnerability to one's living environment or unmet needs. Regardless of etiology, they often can be disturbing to the individual him/herself, family members, and/or health professionals. Also, if left untreated, BPSD can heighten risk for more rapid cognitive decline, hospitalization, functional disability and/or relocation, and caregiver distress. Thus, it is important to prevent BPSD and to reduce or mitigate symptoms if they do occur. As numerous factors may contribute to any given behavior, occupational

Table 6.1 Allowable adaptations to Tailored Activity Program (TAP)

• Translation of materials into different languages
• Training of different care partners including but limited to nurse assistants, home health aides, volunteers, recreational therapists
• Providing additional sessions with the caregiver alone to offer more education, discuss care challenges
• Having another health professional be trained in TAP and offer it under the supervision or in consultation with an occupational therapist
• Having the occupational therapist conduct the assessment phase and another provider implement the activities under guidance from the occupational therapist
• Using assessment tools that differ from those used in the original studies as long as all domains are assessed

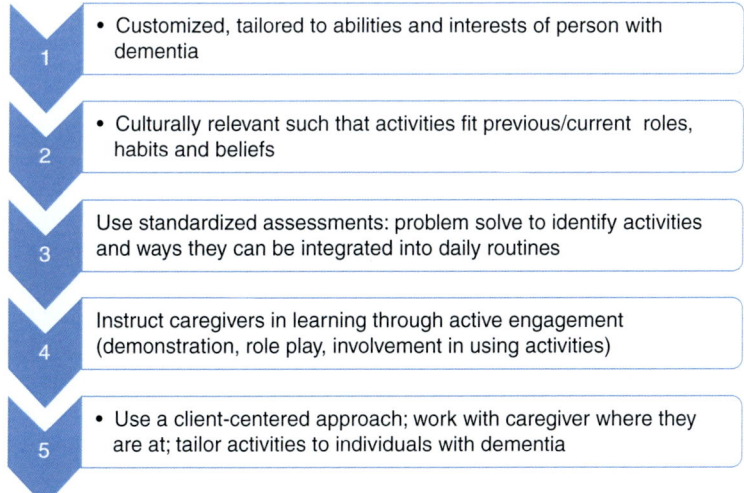

1. • Customized, tailored to abilities and interests of person with dementia

2. • Culturally relevant such that activities fit previous/current roles, habits and beliefs

3. Use standardized assessments: problem solve to identify activities and ways they can be integrated into daily routines

4. Instruct caregivers in learning through active engagement (demonstration, role play, involvement in using activities)

5. • Use a client-centered approach; work with caregiver where they are at; tailor activities to individuals with dementia

Fig. 6.5 Principles for the application of the Tailored Activity Program (TAP)

therapists can have a critical role in its treatment. One program currently being translated for use in a variety of counties and care settings is the TAP program that draws upon competencies of occupational therapists. TAP represents a critical paradigm shift in the way we care for persons living with dementia: it identifies abilities (not just deficits), it designs activities to match intrinsic interest and abilities, and it is a vehicle for illustrating to caregivers what a person can do and what type of support they may need. As an efficacious approach, we recommend it be integrated into traditional occupational therapy practices with persons living with dementia.

6.6 Multi-Sensory Approach in Nursing Homes: Point of View

The concept of multisensory approaches for older adults has been a core aspect of care since the 1980s following developmental work by Hulsegge and Verheul [50]. This initial concept was designed for adults with profound learning disabilities and was used extensively as a leisure activity to increase engagement and wellbeing. The concept used everyday sensory objects such as mobiles, musical instruments, and fabrics to stimulate the senses in a non-directive manner. The potential of such a sensory approach with other client groups soon became apparent and purpose built sensory environments to meet the specific needs of older people have become commonplace. Despite early adoption by many care home facilities, the use of multisensory environments for older adults has been much discussed. In particular, the limited evidence available, lack of appropriate assessment to determine the sensory needs of older adults, and the lack of guidance of how to facilitate a sensory session have resulted in many multisensory environments to be unused despite promising research evidence.

6.6.1 Evidence Underpinning the Use of Multisensory Environments for Older Adults

Research exploring the efficacy of multisensory environments was resisted initially by designers of these spaces as it was felt that formal evaluation would distract from the opportunity for fun and social engagement [50]. Consequently, initial work focused on the aesthetic qualities of the environment and reports of user's enjoyment [51, 52]. Research with older people attempted to focus more on the effect of multisensory environments on mood and behavior, functional performance, and staff/resident interaction. While outcomes have been largely positive, small samples sizes and assessment tools with limited sensitivity have made it difficult for clinicians and care homes to determine the value of the intervention. Table 6.2 illustrates a sample of studies that have explored the use of multisensory environments with older adults.

Although many of the studies listed in Table 6.2 suggest multisensory environments influence mood and behavior, the delivery of the intervention is often unclear.

Table 6.2 Studies exploring the uses of multisensory environments with older adults

Authors	Aim of study	Participants	Assessment	Outcome
Collier et al. [53]	RCT longitudinal, between group Effect of MSE on functional performance	$N = 50$ Mod/severe dementia	Function: AMPS	Significant improvement in functional skills
Maseda et al. [54]	RCT controlled longitudinal, between group; 2xwk sessions for 30 min for 16 weeks, 8 week follow up Effect of MSE on mood, behavior, heart rate, and SpO$_2$	$N = 30$ Mild to severe dementia	Dementia: GDS Pulse oximeters Mood and behavior: Interact	Improved mood and behavior, decreased heart rate, increased SpO$_2$
Maseda et al. [55]	RCT controlled longitudinal, between group; 2xwk sessions for 30 min for 16 weeks, 8 week follow up Effect of MSE on emotion, cognition, function, and agitation	$N = 30$ Mild to severe dementia	Agitation: CMAI Behavior: NPI Cognition: MMSE Function: Barthel index	Reduction in agitation, improved behavior, maintenance of cognition, maintenance of function
Sánchez et al. [56]	RCT pilot between group; two 30-min weekly sessions over 16 weeks. Effect of MSE on mood, agitation, and cognitive status	$N = 32$ Severe dementia	Agitation: CMAI Behavior: NPI Mood: CSDD Cognition: SMMSE	Reduction in agitation, improved behavior, improvement in mood, maintenance of cognition
Collier et al. [27]	Qualitative study To explore concept of MSEs from a user perspective, to study aesthetic and functional qualities, to identify barriers to staff engagement	$N = 16$ care homes	Semi-structured interviews	Preferred equipment predominantly stimulated vision and touch. Staff did not know what to do in the room, good for people in the later stages of the disease, reduces anxiety, can include relatives and care staff

MSE multisensory environment, *AMPS* assessment of motor and process skills, *GDS* global dementia scale, *CMAI* Cohen-Mansfield agitation inventory, *MMSE* mini mental state examination, *NPI* neuropsychiatric inventory, *CSDD* Cornell scale for depression in dementia, *SMMSE* severe mini mental state examination

Studies give little guidance on how to assess the individual or how to establish a multisensory environment for older adults. However, study discussions suggest that the strength of multisensory environments appears to be in the provision of an enriched sensory experience through discrete stimulation without the distraction of the everyday environment. The sensory environment does not place heavy cognitive demand on the individual and can be adapted to create a "just right" challenge for the individual. Studies focusing on the design qualities of the multisensory environment give more guidance particularly in relation to the installation of multisensory environments in care home settings. These design studies have illustrated the need for sensory equipment that is accessible for older adults with sensory impairments, can be used in different areas of the care home, and can be used alongside everyday familiar objects.

6.6.2 Assessment

A number of assessment tools are available that provide baseline data regarding the sensory needs of people with dementia. In particular, the Adult Sensory Profile [57] (ASP) provides an understanding of the sensory processing threshold of the individual. The tool determines the threshold at which an individual may respond to sensory stimulation they are exposed to in the everyday environment, and their behavioral response to that threshold. For example, whether an individual responds to low or high level stimulus and whether their response is to actively manage their response or to remain passive. These behaviors are determined by four categories (Table 6.3):

- high threshold to sensory input with activity management strategies—Sensory seeker
- high threshold to sensory input with passive management strategies—Low registration
- low threshold to sensory input with active management strategies—Sensory avoider
- low threshold to sensory input with passive management strategies—Sensory sensitive

Table 6.3 Model of sensory processing [57]

Behavior		Passive	Active
Sensory threshold	Low	Low registration *Expected physiological response to sensation is a weak response* (due to high threshold) and *quick habituation* (due to accordance behavior that continues to limit response)	Sensory seeker *Expected physiological response to sensation is a weak response* (due to high threshold) and *slow habituation* (due to counteract behavior that pursues sensation)
	High	Sensory sensitive *Expected physiological response to sensation is strong response* (due to low threshold) with *slow habituation* (due to accordance behavior that involves a sustained recognition of available sensation)	Sensory avoider *Expected physiological response to sensation is a strong response* (due to low threshold) with *quick habituation* (due to counteract behavior that withdraws from sensation)

The ASP is a 60 item sensory history questionnaire which is designed to be completed by the individual although caregivers and families can also complete the form. It is validated for use with adolescents and adults between the ages of 16 years and 65 years and older. Items in the questionnaire are rated on a five point Likert scale (1 = seldom, 5 = frequently). Results are analyzed with reference age categories and reported responses to everyday activities.

Other such assessment tools which more explicitly explore sensory processing include the Adult/Adolescent Sensory History (ASH) which also addresses aspects of modulation and discrimination of sensory inputs, postural control, praxis, and social-emotional skills [58]. The ASH is a 163 item questionnaire that can be completed by the individual or a caregiver. It has been validated for use with adolescents and adults between the ages of 13 years to 98 years although predominantly with individuals with learning disabilities. Items in the questionnaire are rated on a five point Likert scale (1 = never, 5 = always), with higher scores suggesting greater levels of dysfunction.

A third assessment tool which considers the over-responsiveness that an individual might experience in everyday activity is the Sensory Over-Responsiveness Scale [59]. This assessment is based on Dunn's model using two behavioral response continua, sensory sensitivity, and sensory avoiding (Table 6.3). Individuals who are sensory over-responsive exhibit exaggerated responses to one or more types of sensory stimuli not normally perceived as threatening, harmful, or noxious. These responses are most commonly experienced through the tactile and auditory sensory systems and affect the individual's ability to engage in everyday activities. The scale is designed in two parts, the sensor assessment, an examiner administered performance scale, and the sensor inventory, a caregiver rating scale.

These sensory processing assessment tools help to determine the level of sensory intensity required in the multisensory environment. Those with a high sensory threshold, who require a higher level of stimulation to maintain levels of arousal to sustain engagement, would require a more multi-modal approach using intense stimulation equipment. Whereas those with a low threshold to sensory stimulation, requiring lower levels of stimulation, would require uni- or bi-modal stimulation using lower intensity equipment. Additionally, these assessments identify sensory preferences in terms of preference for visual, auditory, tactile, taste, smell, movement input. These assessments also help with the construction of the multisensory session by focusing on preferred sensations.

A final assessment of use in constructing a sensory session in a multisensory environment is the Pool Activity Level Occupational Profiling Tool (PAL) [60]. This assessment tool is accessible for carer staff, carers, and family members, and determines how to construct an activity given the cognitive level the individual is functioning. The assessment asks a series of questions about activities that the individual engages in which are rated at the "planned," "exploratory," "sensory," or "reflex" level. These levels reflect levels of cognitive functioning. Once a predominant level is identified then guidance is given on how to construct an activity session. The PAL gives specific guidance on how to run a sensory session in a multisensory environment.

6.6.3 Running a Multisensory Environment Session in a Care Home

Once a sensory assessment has been undertaken the sensory session can be constructed. Guidance from the sensory assessments and the PAL can be used together to determine the items of sensory equipment to be used, the introduction to the session, the facilitation of engagement in the sensory activity, the role of the facilitator during the session, the length of the session, and the conclusion of the session. Those with a high sensory threshold would benefit from a more multisensory experience using equipment to stimulate two or more senses at any one time. The stimulation can also be more intense to trigger a response, for example, the use of more upbeat music, projectors with a reminiscent theme or simulating aromas (citrus fragrance) (Fig. 6.6).

Those with a low sensory threshold would benefit from a more uni-sensory experience possibly of a lower intensity. A singular sensory item may be used based on the individuals sensory preference and used as a point of focus, for example, a fiber optic spray or music with a slow regular rhythm.

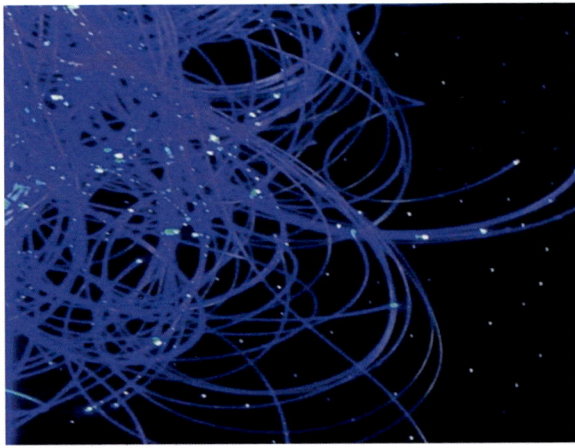

Consideration also needs to be given to whether the multisensory session is to increase levels of arousal and engagement or to reduce levels of arousal, for example reduce levels of anxiety in order to increase engagement. A session to increase levels of arousal might include music with different tempos and rhythm, themed projector images, unfamiliar tactile items, and citrus aromas. A session to reduce levels of anxiety might include a personal choice of music with a tempo of 70 beats a minute or less, relaxing aromas such as lavender, fiber optic spray, and a vibrating cushion.

Multisensory environment sessions can include more than one individual but those sharing a session should have similar sensory needs and be at a similar cognitive level as determined by the PAL. Those with a low cognitive level such as those at the more severe end of a disease spectrum would benefit from a one-to-one interaction with the facilitator in order to accommodate their short attention spans and

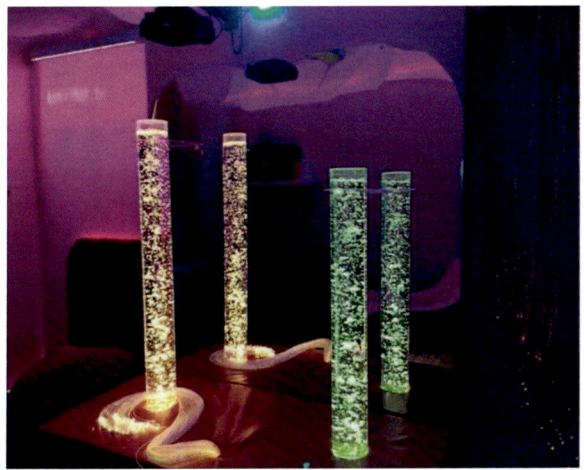

Fig. 6.6   Stimulating multisensory environment. (Author's own picture)

low arousal levels. One-to-one interaction with these individuals also allows the facilitator to be responsive to the subtle indicators of engagement or disengagement that an individual might display.

6.6.4   The Environment

Establishing a multisensory environment can be achieved regardless of budget and space available. Bespoke environments can be created using purpose designed equipment in an exclusive space [61].A number of companies will offer in-house design offering equipment that is suitable for older people. These bespoke options are also available as corner units that can be positioned in general living areas or a sensory trolley that can be set up wherever the sensory session needs to happen such as a bedroom or quiet space. However, these options are costly and multisensory environments are often more successful when they include more familiar items that older people identify with. For example, a basket full of scarves made of different materials (wool, silk, cotton) can provoke engagement, reminiscence, and interaction. A balance between nature and more technical equipment can also make a multisensory environment feel more welcoming for individuals with cognitive impairment who might find the more traditional multisensory environment overwhelming. For example, a sheep skin rug over the chair or an indoor water feature alongside an optic spray.

While dedicated space for a multisensory environment is desirable, the multisensory potential of all environments should be considered. A bathroom may be transformed into a multisensory experience by adjustment to the lighting (using softer lighting, switching off overhead strip lighting), using aroma diffusers or scented bath products, inclusion of the individual's preferred music, and different textured washing clothes (rough loofah, sponge, soft wash cloth). Being in the garden can be a multisensory experience with different scented and textured plants, wind chimes, different textured walk ways (grass, gravel, tarmac), and colorful wind ornaments. Multisensory opportunities should be considered throughout the whole environment.

In conclusion, establishing a multisensory environment or space for older people has the potential to address issues such as mental health, disengagement, and ill-being. Multisensory environments are accessible for all older people regardless of physical or psychological limitations and can be set up regardless of the space available. However, multisensory environments are only a tool so a robust assessment needs to be undertaken to identify what the sensory needs of the individual are and to help design a successful multisensory session.

Key Messages

1. People with dementia living in nursing home can be engaged in meaningful activities at any level of cognitive impairment or challenging behavior until they respond to the environment and express pleasure.
2. Progressive cognitive impairment implies the use of more simple activities, divided into one or two step type with eventually use of sensory cues, to support initiating and sequencing. In nursing home occupational therapist's skill is able to comprehend the complex interaction between cognitive, functional disabilities, and environment and he is able to plan a client centered approach that includes psychosocial interventions, personal interests, and values.
3. In case of challenging behaviors in NH it is most important to consider a collaborative and integrated care model with all professionals. Occupational therapist can help team to analyze the characterization of challenging behavior and the context in which they occur and develop a tailored activity program in a supportive context.
4. Occupational therapist plays an important role in supporting formal and informal caregiver to understand the disease and its manifestations and implications. He can train NH staff and caregivers in the best way to approach and communicate with people with dementia and how to prevent and manage behavioral and psychological symptoms.

    People with dementia at any stage of disease can benefit of a multisensory environment and multisensory activities. Multisensory experience includes lighting, aroma diffusers, music, touch experience. A facilitator can be useful to adapt the correct stimulus respect of resident's interests, sensory and cognitive deficit.

References

1. Ballard C, O'Brien J, James I, Mynt P, Lana M, Potkins D, et al. Quality of life for people with dementia living in residential and nursing home care: the impact of performance on activities of daily living, behavioral and psychological symptoms, language skills, and psychotropic drugs. Int Psychogeriatr. 2001;13(1):93–106.

2. Habiger T, Husebø BS, Ballard C, Slettebo DD, Flo E, Testad I, et al. The effect of a multicomponent intervention on quality of life in residents of nursing homes: a randomized controlled trial (COSMOS). J Am Med Dir Assoc. 2019;20(3):330–9.
3. Maenhout A, Cornelis E, Van de Velde D, Desmet V, Gorus E, VanMalderen L, et al. The relationship between quality of life in nursing home and personal, organizational, activity-related factors and social satisfaction: a cross-sectional study with multiple linear regression analyses. Aging Ment Health. 2019. https://doi.org/10.1080/13607863.2019.1571014 [Epub ahead of print].
4. Brooker DJ, Woolley RJ. Enriching opportunities for people living with dementia: the development of a blueprint for a sustainable activity-based model. Aging Ment Health. 2007;11(4):371–83.
5. Kolanowski Ann BL. Prescribing activities that engage passive residents. An innovative method. J Gerontol Nurs. 2008;34(1):13–8.
6. Kitwood T. Dementia reconsidered: the person comes first, Rethinking aging. Buckingham: Open University Press; 1997.
7. Livingston G, Kelly L, Lewis-Holmes E, Baio G, Morris S, Patel N, et al. Non-pharmacological interventions for agitation in dementia: systematic review of randomised controlled trials. Br J Psychiatry. 2014;205:436–42.
8. Kim SK, Park M. Effectiveness of person-centered care on people with dementia: a systematic review and meta-analysis. Clin Interv Aging. 2017;12:381–97.
9. Romeo R, Zala D, Knapp M, Orrell M, Fossey J, Ballard C. Improving the quality of life of care home residents with dementia: cost-effectiveness of an optimized intervention for residents with clinically significant agitation in dementia. Alzheimers Dement. 2019;15(2):282–91.
10. Koren MJ. Person-centered care for nursing home residents: the culture-change movement. Health Aff. 2010;29:312–7.
11. Hermer L, Doll GA, Cornelison L, Poey JL, Stone RI, Drake PN, Kaup ML. Person-centered care as facilitated by Kansas' PEAK 2.0 Medicaid pay-for-performance program and nursing home resident clinical outcomes. Innov Aging. 2018;2(3):1–12.
12. Bradshaw SA, Playford ED, Riazi A. Living well in care homes: a systematic review of qualitative studies. Age Ageing. 2012;41:429–40.
13. Jones M. Gentle care: changing the experience of Alzheimer's disease in a positive way. Burnaby BC: Moyra Jones Resources; 1996.
14. Hall GR, Buckwalter KC. Progressively lowered stress threshold: a conceptual model for care of adults with Alzheimer's disease. Arch Psychiatr Nurs. 1987;1:399–406.
15. Gage H, Hurley MV, Anderson L, Grant R, Koskela SA, Clarke N, et al. Active residents in care homes (ARCH): study protocol to investigate the implementation and outcomes of a whole-systems activity programme in residential care homes for older people. Physiotherapy. 2015;103(1):113–20.
16. Graff MJL, Vernooij-Dassen MJM, Thijssen M, Dekker J, Hoefnagels WHL, Rikkert MGMO. Community based occupational therapy for patients with dementia and their care givers: randomised controlled trial. Br Med J. 2006;333(7580):1196–9.
17. Graff MJL, Adang EMM, Vernooij-Dassen MJM, Dekker J, Jönsson L, Thijssen M, et al. Community occupational therapy for older patients with dementia and their care givers: cost effectiveness study. BMJ. 2008;336(7636):134–8.
18. Manni B, Federzoni L, Lanzoni A, Garzetta G, Graff M, Fabbo A. Occupational therapy in special respite care: a new multicomponent model for challenging behavior in people with dementia. Geriatr Care. 2018;4:7649.
19. Regier NG, Hodgson NA, Gitlin LN. Characteristics of activities for persons with dementia at the mild, moderate, and Severe Stages. Gerontologist. 2017;57(5):987–97.
20. Lima-Silva TB, Bahia VS, Carvalho VA, Guimarães HC, Caramelli P, Balthazar ML, et al. Neuropsychiatric symptoms, caregiver burden and distress in behavioral-variant frontotemporal dementia and Alzheimer's disease. Dement Geriatr Cogn Disord. 2015;40:268–75.
21. Costello H, Walsh S, Cooper C, Livingston G. A systematic review and meta-analysis of the prevalence and associations of stress and burnout among staff in long-term care facilities for people with dementia. Int Psychogeriatr. 2019;31(8):1203–16.

22. Fossey J, Ballard C, Juszczak E, James I, Alder N, Jacoby R, Howard R. Effect of enhanced psychosocial care on antipsychotic use in nursing home residents with severe dementia: cluster randomised trial. Br Med J. 2006;332(7544):756–8.
23. Testad I, Corbett A, Aarsland D, Lexow KO, Fossey J, Woods B, Ballard C. The value of personalized psychosocial interventions to address behavioral and psychological symptoms in people with dementia living in care home settings: a systematic review. Int Psychogeriatr. 2014;26(7):1083–98.
24. Travers C, Brooks D, Hines S, O'Reilly M, McMaster M, He W, MacAndrew M, Fielding E, Karlsson L, Beattie E. Effectiveness of meaningful occupation interventions for people living with dementia in residential aged care: a systematic review. JBI Database System Rev Implement Rep. 2016;14(12):163–225.
25. Ballard C, Corbett A, Orrell M, Williams G, Moniz-Cook E, Romeo R, et al. Impact of person-centred care training and person-centred activities on quality of life, agitation, and antipsychotic use in people with dementia living in nursing homes: a cluster-randomised controlled trial. PLoS Med. 2018;15(2):e1002500.
26. Staal JA, Sacks A, Matheis R, Collier L, Calia T, Hanif H, Kofman ES. The effects of Snoezelen (multi-sensory behavior therapy) and psychiatric care on agitation, apathy, and activities of daily living in dementia patients on a short term geriatric psychiatric inpatient unit. Int J Psychiatry Med. 2007;37(4):357–70.
27. Collier L, Jakob A. The multisensory environment (MSE) in dementia care: examining its role and quality from a user perspective. HERD. 2017;10(5):39–51.
28. Gitlin L, Verrier Piersol C, Hodgson N, Marx K, Roth DL, Johnston D, Samus Q, Pizzi L, Jutkowitz E, Lyketsos CG. Reducing neuropsychiatric symptoms in persons with dementia and associated burden in family caregivers using tailored activities: design and methods of a randomized clinical trial. Contemp Clin Trials. 2016;49:92–102.
29. Gitlin LN, Arthur P, Piersol C, Hessels V, Wu SS, Dai Y, Mann WC. Targeting behavioral symptoms and functional decline in dementia: a randomized clinical trial. J Am Geriatr Soc. 2018;66(2):339–45.
30. Gitlin LN, Marx KA, Alonzi D, Kvedar T, Moody J, Trahan M, Van Haitsma K. Feasibility of the tailored activity program for hospitalized (TAP-H) patients with behavioral symptoms. Gerontologist. 2017;57(3):575–84.
31. Fraker J, Kales HC, Blazek M, Kavanagh J, Gitlin LN. The role of the occupational therapist in the management of neuropsychiatric symptoms of dementia in clinical settings. Occup Ther Health Care. 2014;28(1):4–20.
32. Gitlin LN, Hodgson N. Better living with dementia: implications for individuals, families, communities and societies. San Diego, CA: Academic Press; 2018.
33. Gitlin LN, Kales HC, Lyketsos CG. Nonpharmacologic management of behavioral symptoms in dementia. JAMA. 2012;308(19):2020–9.
34. Miyamoto Y, Tachimori H, Ito H. Formal caregiver burden in dementia: impact of behavioral and psychological symptoms of dementia and activities of daily living. Geriatr Nurs. 2010;31(4):246–53.
35. Matsumoto N, Ikeda M, Fukuhara R, Shinagawa S, Ishikawa T, Mori T, et al. Caregiver burden associated with behavioral and psychological symptoms of dementia in elderly people in the local community. Dement Geriatr Cogn Disord. 2007;23:219–24.
36. Arthur PB, Gitlin LN, Kairalla J, Mann W. Relationship between the number of behavioral symptoms in dementia and caregiver distress: what is the tipping point? Int Psychogeriatr. 2018;30(8):1099–107.
37. Gitlin LN, Winter L, Dennis MP, Hodgson N, Hauck WW. Targeting and managing behavioral symptoms in individuals with dementia: a randomized trial of a nonpharmacological intervention. J Am Geriatr Soc. 2010;58(8):1465–74.
38. Kales HC, Gitlin LN, Lyketsos CG. Prevention, assessment and management of behavioral and psychological symptoms of dementia: the need for a tailored patient- and caregiver-centered approach. BMJ. 2015;350:h369.

39. Hodgson N, Gitlin LN, Winter L, Hauck WW. Caregiver's perceptions of the relationship of pain to behavioral and psychiatric symptoms in older community residing adults with dementia. Clin J Pain. 2014;30(5):421–7.
40. Hodgson NA, Gitlin LN, Winter L, Czekanski K. Undiagnosed illness and neuropsychiatric behaviors in community-residing older adults with dementia. Alzheimer Dis Assoc Disord. 2011;25(2):109–15.
41. Kales HC, Zivin K, Kim H, et al. Trends in antipsychotic use in dementia 1999–2007. Arch Gen Psychiatry. 2011;68(2):190–7.
42. Sink KM, Holden KF, Yaffe K. Pharmacological treatment of neuropsychiatric symptoms of dementia: a review of the evidence. J Am Med Assoc. 2005;293(5):596–608.
43. Maust DT, Kim M, Chiang C, Kales HC. Association of the Centers for Medicare & Medicaid Services' National Partnership to Improve Dementia Care with the use of Antipsychotics and Other Psychotropics in Long-term Care in the United States from 2009 to 2014. JAMA Intern Med. 2018;178(5):640–7.
44. Kales HC, Gitlin LN, Lyketsos CG, Detroit expert panel on the assessment and management of the neuropsychiatric symptoms of dementia. Management of neuropsychiatric symptoms of dementia in clinical settings: recommendations from a multidisciplinary expert panel. J Am Geriatr Soc. 2014;62(4):762–9.
45. Odenheimer G, Borson S, Sanders AE, Swain-Eng RJ, Kyomen HH, Tierney S, Johnson J. Quality improvement in neurology: dementia management quality measures. J Am Geriatr Soc. 2014;62(3):558–61.
46. Gitlin LN, Piersol CV, Hodgson N, Marx K, Roth D, Johnson D, Samus Q, Pizzi L, Jutkowitz E, Lyketos CG. Reducing neuropsychiatric symptoms in persons with dementia and associated burden in family caregivers using tailored activities: design and methods of a randomized clinical trial. Contemp Clin Trials. 2016;49:92–102.
47. Gitlin LN, Winter L, Earland TV, Herge EA, Chernett NL, Piersol CV, Burke JP. The tailored activity program (TAP) to reduce behavioral symptoms in individuals with dementia: feasibility, acceptability, and replication potential. The Gerontologist. 2009;49:428–39.
48. Novielli M, Machado SCC, Lima GB, et al. Effects of the tailored activity program in Brazil (TAP-BR) for persons with dementia: a randomized pilot trial. Alzheimer Dis Assoc Disord. 2018;32(4):339–45.
49. Gitlin LN, Piersol CV. A Caregiver's guide to dementia: using activity and other strategies to prevent, reduce, and manage behavioral symptoms. Philadelphia, PA: Camino Books, Inc; 2014.
50. Hulsegge J, Verheul A. Snoezelen. Chesterfield: Rompa UK Publications; 1987.
51. Haggar L, Hutchinson R. Snoezelen: an approach to the provision of a leisure resource for people with profound and multiple handicaps. Mental Handicap. 1991;19(2):51–5.
52. Hutchinson R, Haggar L. The development and evaluation of a Snoezelen leisure resource for people with profound and multiple handicaps. In: Kewin J, editor. The Whittington Hall Snoezelen project. Chesterfield: North Derbyshire Health Authority; 1991.
53. Collier L, McPherson K, Ellis-Hill C, Staal J, Bucks R. Multisensory stimulation to improve functional performance in moderate to severe dementia—interim results. Am J Alzheimers Dis Other Dement. 2010;25(8):698–703.
54. Maseda A, Sánchez A, Marante M, González-Abraldes I, Buján A, Millan-Calenti JC. Effects of multisensory stimulation on a sample of institutionalized elderly people with dementia diagnosis: a controlled longitudinal trial. Am J Alzheimers Dis Other Dement. 2014;29(5):463–73.
55. Maseda A, Sánchez A, Marante M, González-Abraldes I, de Labra C, Millan-Calenti JC. Multisensory stimulation on mood, behavior, and biomedical parameters in people with dementia: is it more effective than conventional one-to-one stimulation? Am J Alzheimers Dis Other Dement. 2014;29:637–47.
56. Sánchez A, Marante-Moar P, Sarabia C, de Labra C, Lorenzo T, Maseda A, Carlos Millan-Calenti J. Multisensory stimulation as an intervention strategy for elderly patients with severe dementia: a pilot randomized controlled trial. Am J Alzheimers Dis Other Dement. 2016;31(4):341–50.

57. Brown C, Tollefson N, Dunn W, Cromwell R, Filion D. The adult sensory profile: measuring patterns of sensory processing. Am J Occup Ther. 2001;55:75–82.
58. May-Benson T. The adult/adolescent sensory history (ASH). Newtown, MA: Spiral Foundation; 2015.
59. Schoen SA, Miller LJ, Green KE. Pilot study of the sensory over-responsivity scales: assessment and inventory. Am J Occup Ther. 2008;62:393–406.
60. Pool J. The Pool activity level (PAL) instrument for occupational profiling. 4th ed. London: Jessica Kinglsey; 2012.
61. Jakob A, Collier L. Sensory design for dementia care – the benefits of textiles. J Text Des Res Pract. 2017;5(2):232–50.

Occupational Therapy and Palliative Care

7

Elena Lucchi, Giovanna Caiata-Olgiati,
Marina Bonomi, and Fabio Cembrani

7.1 Introduction: The Philosophy of Palliative Care

The philosophy of palliative care was born in a much older historical time since the era in which, despite the prodigious advances of modern medicine, the need for medical science to move from the concept of healing at all costs to the more realistic attention to the "total care" of the sick person. Already in the Middle Ages, throughout Europe, there were places, called hospices, deputies for the reception of the destitute, the sick and those dying. The sick were cared for and treated, physically and spiritually, and accompanied with in the final journey of life. One of the most famous was the Hôtel-Dieu de Beaune (France).

The concept of palliation, in the sense of a charitable and merciful approach, has always existed. It is from the Latin word *pallium*, the veil used to cover the wearer, which derives the meaning of "to palliate" in medicine, understood as covering, treating the symptom of the disease and not its cause. An ancient role when illness and death constituted an essential element of the vision of life of the human being,

E. Lucchi (✉)
Department of Rehabilitation and Unit of Palliative Care, Teresa Camplani Foundation, Cremona, Italy

G. Caiata-Olgiati
University of Applied Sciences of Italian Switzerland – SUPSI, Manno, Switzerland

Caribù Occupational Therapy Center in Biasca, Biasca, Switzerland
e-mail: giovanna.caiata@supsi.ch

M. Bonomi
Neuromotor Rehabilitation of ASST Crema, Cremona, Italy

Occupational Therapy University of Milan, Milan, Italy

F. Cembrani
Department of Legal Medicine, Provincial Company for Health Services of Trento, Trento, Italy
e-mail: fabio.cembrani@apss.tn.it

© Springer Nature Switzerland AG 2020
C. Pozzi et al. (eds.), *Occupational Therapy for Older People*,
https://doi.org/10.1007/978-3-030-35731-3_7

but that it was necessary to rediscover and reconfirm when scientific advances have pushed the human being to the illusion of a victory over death and illnesses. Thus medicine, in an attempt to hide or oppose its inevitable failures, has increasingly eliminated the palliative from its tasks, leading to a tendency towards therapeutic obstinacy, not seen in negative terms, but as a natural consequence of a medicine mistakenly seen as omnipotent and infallible.

Fortunately, around the 1950s there was a rapprochement with issues such as death. In 1956 Herman Feifel, Karl Junge, and Robert Kastenbaum organized the "Conference on the problem of death" from which emerged the concept of the culture of good death with the aim of guaranteeing an end that is as dignified as possible to people with incurable diseases [1]. In the 1960s John Bowlby and Colin Murray Parkes worked together to understand the grieving process, analyzing it from the perspective of attachment theory [2]. In 1967, the St. Christopher's Hospice was founded in London, founded by Cicely Saunders and universally recognized as the first modern hospice that embodied the characteristics of the philosophy of the hospice movement: a welcoming and familiar environment, continuous assistance based on a multidimensional approach to symptoms causes discomfort. From the experience of the St. Christopher, starting from the revolutionary concept of total pain, modern palliative care is born which shifts the focus of the intervention on the identification and satisfaction of the needs of the sick person and no longer on the mere, even if fundamental, pain therapy. Starting from this model, in England and in other 90 countries of the world the first Hospices are beginning to be born and the adhesions to the palliative care model.

In 2002, the World Health Organization defined palliative care as "an approach that improves the quality of life and patient and treatment of pain and other problems, physical, psychosocial, and spiritual" (WHO Definition of Palliative Care. Available at: www.who.int/cancer/palliative/definition/en) [3]. Palliative care:

- provides relief from pain and other distressing symptoms;
- affirms life and regards dying as a normal process;
- intends neither to hasten or postpone death;
- integrates the psychological and spiritual aspects of patient care;
- offers a support system to help patient's live as actively as possible until death;
- offers a support system to help the family cope during the patients illness and in their own bereavement;
- uses a team approach to address the needs of patients and their families, including bereavement counseling, if indicated;
- will enhance quality of life, and may also positively influence the course of illness;
- is applicable early in the course of illness, in conjunction with other therapies that are intended to prolong life, such as chemotherapy or radiation therapy, and includes those investigations needed to better understand and manage distressing clinical complications.

The WHO recognizes palliative care among global fundamental strategies for universal health coverage. However, in the world palliative care is a denied right for over 36 million people (Quotidianosanità.it 18 August 2017).

According to the WHO Global Atlas of Palliative Care (2014), only 20 WHO countries (8.6%) have advanced hospital palliative care services from the point of view of basic supply, with the following characteristics:

- development of a palliative care activity in a wide range of situations;
- complete provision of all types of palliative care by multiple services;
- broad awareness of palliative care by health professionals, local communities, and society in general;
- availability of morphine and all other strong medications to relieve pain;
- substantial impact of palliative care on public health policy;
- development of recognized education centers;
- academic links with universities;
- existence of a national palliative care association.

Australia, Austria, Belgium, Canada, France, Germany, Hong Kong, Iceland, Ireland, Italy, Japan, Norway, Poland, Romania, Singapore, Sweden, Switzerland, Uganda, the United Kingdom, and the USA are part of this group.

According to the Global Atlas of Palliative Care at the End of Life of the WHO (2014) [4] most adults who require palliative care die from cardiovascular diseases (38.5%), and cancer (34%), followed by people with chronic respiratory diseases (10.3%) (Fig. 7.1), pathologies at high frequencies in the elderly population.

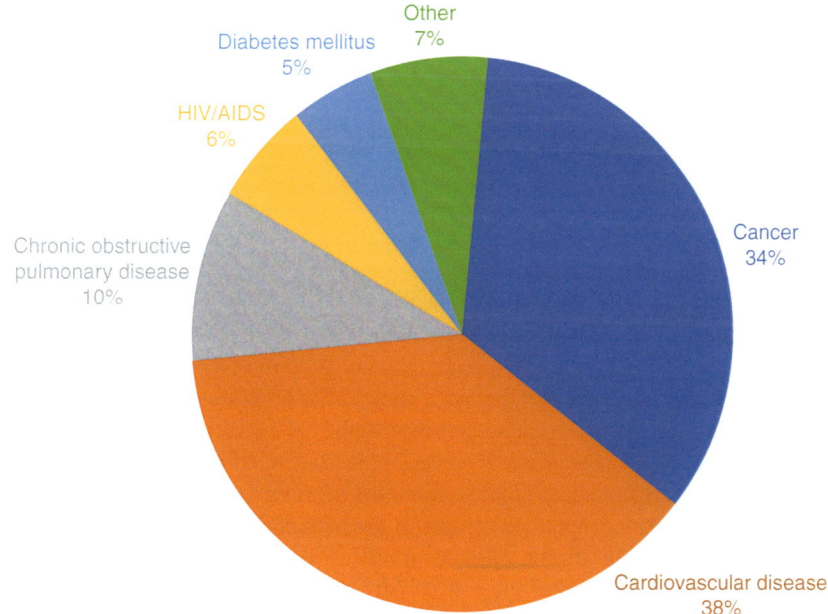

Fig. 7.1 Need for access to palliative care for adults, based on the pathology (modified from: Worldwide Palliative Care Alliance World Health Organization. 2014 Global Atlas of Palliative Care at the End of Life) [4]

Worldwide, over 20 million people are estimated to require palliative care at the end of life every year. The majority (69%) are adults over 60 years old and only 6% are children.

It is fundamental, therefore, that the palliative approach includes as much as possible all the care resources available, including the occupational therapy can play a fundamental role in achieving the goals that palliative care aims to achieve.

7.2   Background: Review of the Literature on Palliative Care and Occupational Therapy

Since occupational therapy is a rehabilitative health profession that promotes health and quality of life through employment, in particular through specific interventions aimed at restoring or preserving the activities of daily life, emerges clearly as such a figure fully belongs to the fundamental ones to reach the goals that palliative care sets for itself.

Achieving a good quality of life is strongly linked to the commitment to pleasant and meaningful activities for the sick person.

The contribution of the occupational therapist in palliative care is therefore to promote the maintenance of pleasant abilities, autonomy and independence, identity and the occupational role of the sick person [5]. In fact, the person who is in the terminal phase can risk seeing his identity weakened, through the loss of the previous role, professional or social.

The occupational therapist, through the interventions on the strengthening of the occupational identity, acts on the sense of self as the primary subject of activity, through the understanding of the motivational drive, of the inclinations, of the sphere of habits.

Working to improve the quality of life of the patient should not be limited to the management of problems closely related to symptoms such as pain, fatigue, dyspnea, but also to the promotion of the centrality of the sick person who must still be able to feel the protagonist of his life, through the possibility to have a role, activity, and possibility to decide for himself.

Despite these assumptions that see the role of occupational therapy as fundamental for people who take advantage of palliative care, there are not many jobs available that investigate the role and effectiveness of such interventions in PC.

Most of the studies are conducted in Anglo-Saxon countries (UK, Australia), where the modern palliative approach originated.

The need to refer to a *theoretical model* of practice in palliative care is fundamental for the occupational therapy intervention that necessarily starts with an evaluation process to define the occupational profile of the patient [6], besides being necessary the use of tools capable of assessing the quality of life to support the intervention of occupational therapy in the practice of palliative care [7]. The occupational therapist must therefore gather information on the occupational profile to try to understand what the significant and relevant occupations are, the daily routine, the interests, the values, and priorities. In addition to this it is essential to know the vision of life and the expectations regarding the death that patients have. It is also essential to be able to interview caregivers, the family, and anyone who has a patient relevance to be helped in defining the patient's preferences and priorities, particularly when it is difficult to identify his desires and goals during the end of life.

The OPHI-II, an instrument of the American model MOHO (Model of Human Occupation), is considered as a valid tool for proceeding with the evaluation of the terminally ill [6]. Studied and developed by Kielhofner in the 1980s, it includes a semi-structured interview that explores the patient's occupational life; three scales that provide an assessment of the patient's occupational identity, his occupational competence, and the impact of the patient's occupational behavior settings; a narration of his life story aimed at capturing the salient qualitative characteristics of the history of occupational life. The strength of this tool, used in palliative care, is the possibility of investigating the cultural, spiritual, and social factors that influence the patient, allowing the OT to gather fundamental information to help the terminal patient understand how to deal with his life and to make new life expectations, albeit limited. For example, the patient might prefer to be dressed by the caregiver, in order to keep his energies to tell and share his story with his loved ones.

MOHO is therefore a model of occupational therapy practice that brings out the possibilities that terminal illness can also offer to the patient, through the modification of their occupational identity and their ability to be engaged in significant occupations [8, 9]. Table 7.1 lists the main factors that influence the quality of life as emerged from the literature [6] and how these find a close correspondence with the objectives of occupational therapy.

The *narration* was by far the most discussed topic in the literature concerning OT in Cunningham [10] argues that occupational therapy is one of the professions that most offers a helping relationship to his patients. The beginning of the occupational therapy process must coincide with the beginning of the therapeutic relationship. The outline of the occupational history of the person taken into care is necessary, regardless of age or the disease from which it is affected [11]. Since the *memory* of us in life is closely related to the transmission of our being to others [12], even in the terminal phase of life the memory we leave can be transmitted through the actions we take and thanks to what we have physically produced in life: memory is therefore closely connected to occupations and to one's own occupational identity, even in the final phase of one's life. The obstacles can be many, especially during the stay in hospice patients can suffer from communication difficulties with the team, feeling unwell. For this reason the narration plays a fundamental role in the patient's approach to the OT (as well as to the whole team) since it has a direct action on improving the quality of life in hospice. The meaning of the narrative lies in the possibility given to patients to give meaning to past experiences and to associate the events of their life by dealing with themes such as values, interests, and spirituality [9]. This narrative necessity, which is very significant in the terminally ill patient, has the ability to redefine its occupational roles within the context (space and current time). The patient's narrative becomes effective only when a relationship is established between patient and occupational therapist, without departing from a client-centered approach [8].

Table 7.1 Factors that influence the quality of life in people in the terminal phase (taken and modified by Pizzi [6])

Factors that influence the quality of life and the quality of health at the end of life	Relationship with occupational therapy
Maintenance of residual abilities and participation in life activities that contribute to quality of life	Occupational therapists believe that continued participation in occupations helps the person to continue his life and that this is fundamental in health and quality of life. Pre-emptively changing occupations to make them accessible and adding new ones to compensate for the loss of old ones prevent isolation and contribute to a sense of self-worth
Maintaining the sense of control contributes to the quality of life	Through participation in daily life occupations that patients consider significant, they can choose, and this gives them a sense of control, identity, and competence
Continuing to contribute to others and remain connected to important relationships contributes to the quality of life	Patient participation in tasks and activities is a primary goal in occupational therapy intervention. Carrying out tasks or activities, such as writing a letter to grandchildren or rewriting their favorite recipes using the social context of the person helps the person feel productive and helps them to stay connected with the people they care about
Continue to seek the meaning of life and live one's spirituality	Occupational therapists recognize spirituality as an important factor for patients. They believe that participation in occupations helps the person to connect with their own sense of life which supports spirituality, well-being, and quality of life. Participation in occupations can combat the sense of unhappiness, ineffectiveness, and renunciation that may arise during the terminal phase of life. Occupational therapists help patients recognize the meaningful occupations in which they want to engage and provide new strategies for continuing to participate

The most common initial approach with a patient in palliative care is of a conversational relational type [5]. In the majority of patients, conversation, a tool adopted by the occupational therapist in a particular way in the geriatric patient and in the terminal patient, is considered a relational situation that creates well-being, as it restores the individual's centrality and self-esteem and addresses the patient's whole parts. Furthermore, the subject who is able to converse makes explicit some emotional, communicative, contractual, and decision-making competences, which often risk weakening or getting lost in the hospitalized patient.

Supporting *participation* in significant activities is another topic widely discussed in the literature and represents one of the main aspects associated with the effectiveness of occupational therapy intervention. The loss of *independence* and roles can be a priority problem with respect to biological death and therefore, occupational therapy can help people to identify new occupational roles and significant new occupations to maintain a good level of self-esteem [13]. Terminal patients are often not actively involved in their occupational nature, but this represents an extremely negative condition [14], in fact the possibility of being able to participate in significant occupations having an imminent death ahead is an option on which everyone should be able to choose, if they wish [15]. Hospices do not have rehabilitation as their goal, but they must necessarily face and work in order to maintain autonomy and independence in patients' lives, eliminating all limitations. These goals are perfectly aligned with the objectives of occupational therapy practice [8].

The Model of Human Occupation—MOHO [11] is useful and searchable for an application in the field of palliative care. Occupations, as they are integrated and conceived in the MOHO model, refer to the interaction between the person and their ability to participate in occupations. This participation takes place in a specific time frame, socio-cultural, or in a specific physical contest [9]. A combined intervention between OT and physiotherapist, in a hospice with terminal cancer patients, has been shown to be effective in decreasing physical fatigue, in significantly increasing its functions and the ability to use new strategies to perform significant occupations [16]. According to Pizzi [6], occupational therapists help patients to relieve them of pain and increase their quality of life, supporting them in participating in daily life occupations that patients consider significant. At the end of one's life, when people have lost their previous occupational roles, their jobs, their performance skills, it becomes necessary to identify and support participation in new and other meaningful occupations. It is therefore important to identify and adopt compensation strategies, which require a specific performance analysis and a possible modification of the physical environment, which can be a support to promote the patient's abilities and participation.

Occupational therapy intervention for a terminal patient may aim to alleviate symptoms that interfere with function and action. Participation in significant occupations for the person not only increases the patient's quality of life, but also acquires an important role in controlling symptoms and pain [17]: patients who pay more attention to participation in significant activities pay less attention to what are the disturbing physical symptoms. The person with a pathology in an advanced state sees his or her life stripped of all its occupations [18]: the occupational therapist intervenes specifically in these areas with the aim of strengthening motivation, the sphere of habits and self-awareness, supporting participation in significant occupations.

Research has shown that participation in occupations at the end of life is essential for maintaining meaningful relationships, for a sense of effectiveness, they have a strong impact on the person's living environment and an important reflection on everyday life [8, 19].

Even in the last phase of their lives, through participation in significant occupations, people can try to continue their history through ways they consider significant, satisfying and achievable [5]. The task of the OT is to modify the requests of the activity, the habits, and routines associated with the occupations to be able to identify which are the most appropriate methods based on the performance capabilities and tolerance of patients and caregivers; all this is necessary in order to allow the person to participate in the significant occupations that emerged [20].

Maintaining contact and control with *relationships* and people is an important issue to consider in occupational therapy with a terminal patient. The OT in the evaluation of environmental and contextual factors must take the person and their social contacts well into consideration to avoid social isolation, a very common condition in patients at the end of life. Carrying out tasks or activities, such as writing a letter to grandchildren or rewriting their favorite recipes to pass on to family members using the social context of the person, helps the person feel productive and helps them to stay connected with the people they care about [6].

In the literature it has emerged how the use of *creative and play activities* is important in the intervention of occupational therapy with a terminal patient. The pleasure and sense of self-esteem increase in family occupations related to leisure and to one's passions [6]. Participation in creative activities helps patients slow down the decline in residual skills and creates new connections with life [21, 22].

Welcoming and supporting *spirituality* is a fundamental aspect of the intervention of occupational therapy in the treatment of the terminally ill. The American Occupational Therapy Association [23] states that occupational therapists recognize spirituality as an important factor for patients: participation in occupations helps the person to connect with their own sense of life that they support spirituality, well-being, quality of life. Hunter [12] reports that the memory of us in life is closely related to the transmission of one's being to others; the memory we leave can be transmitted through actions and through what was physically produced in life. In both cases, this memory is closely connected to the occupations and their own occupational identity that people experience during their lives. Occupational therapy intervention can engage the patient in tasks or activities that focus on the perception it can have of itself in this stage of its life [8]. Just as in the terminally ill the sense of acting dumb, sensations, and volition change, which can significantly affect occupational performance, especially in the sphere of spirituality.

For Hammillet al. [20] the most widely used and valid approaches by Australian occupational therapists are only compensatory approaches, approaches related to the adaptation of performance and the environment, and approaches aimed at maintaining residual abilities. The effectiveness of the occupational therapy intervention in palliative care has been demonstrated in several studies and does not differ from the classic approach of occupational therapy in other areas, as well as being extremely linked to the identification of the activities that are part of the occupational history, and that this information must necessarily be obtained in a rapid time, even more so in an area such as palliative care [8]. A common aspect that emerged in the literature analysis is the need for more specific training on CP by the OT, as well as a greater attention to the evaluation process of interventions, a fundamental aspect to be able to produce valid, repeatable, and significant scientific evidence. Although the theoretical assumptions exist for retaining the central OT in PCs as well as supporting evidence for such interventions, even if limited to a few studies, the spread of this approach is extremely limited, compared to the potential.

7.3   The Application of Occupational Therapy in Palliative Care: An Example

In this section we will show how palliative care is not only represented by terminal care in people with oncological diseases: even in the geriatric field, palliative care can be a long-term illness intervention, with reality of life that can still be very intense and diversified. Not all the elderly needs palliative care: some live without particular problems taking advantage of his own autonomy and still being independently at home by fulfilling their tasks and occupations in a well-defined role, in a good or fair state of health. When, on the other hand, the elderly person presents fragility and comorbidity, falling within the patient identification criteria of palliative care (Flowchart for the identification of a patient's clinical care in a palliative unit of the "Istituto Oncologico della Svizzera Italiana"),[1] we begin to consider a change of perspective, involving specific care, in looking after persons, to deal with the dignity and respect of the daily efforts and the renunciations to which people are forced.

In the occupational therapy professional practice, the life story of the person is always present; not only for what she has done, but also for how she has been able to face difficulties in situations, identifying personal resources, seeking and finding solutions, asking for help, and finding energy in front of her diseases. That disease which, as described in Ardia and Caiata-Olgiati [24], "modifies our body, making it suffer, weakening it and sometimes mutilating it. The person, progressively or suddenly, finds herself with a different body than she was used to living with. The projection of herself in the space and in the time changes, the physical capacities are altered, the look that she carries about herself, changes." It is an illness that produce, in addition to generalized suffering (total pain), anger, sadness, fears, anguish, rebellion and which exacerbates the deep "why?" through questions of meaning, sense, fundamental inquiry about life and death. The disease plunges the person into the phases of bereavement, as defined by Kübler Ross [25]. The occupational therapist, therefore, also has the task of helping the other person to face life in the illness, through the mourning of the loss of health, to transform it slowly into an occasion, an opportunity to discover a new way of being and doing.

Below is reported, as example, the case of a patient taken care by an occupational therapist within a palliative care approach in the Swiss Italian territory.

Mrs. A., 84 years old, use to be teacher in a primary school, had always lived alone, involved in different types of volunteering and responsibilities, a very independent person in everything she has done, whom still drove a car. Following a cervical surgery, she had a stroke and she awaked hemiplegic and completely dependent. She was in a devastating shock, as this state was not contemplated as a possibility of risk!

She immediately started an acute rehabilitation in a specialist clinic, but seeing that, in the following months, no significant changes were noticed, Mrs. A. demoralized further and further, and she begun to shut down on herself, and in a short time

---

[1] https://www.eoc.ch/dms/site-eoc/documenti/pallclick/Cura-del-Paziente/Criteri-Identificazione-PZ-CP-spiegazioni.

she was completely depressed, often lying in bed or sitting in wheelchair, silently angry. After 6 months of intensive rehabilitation she had not achieved any improvement or well-being, on the contrary, she was even further plunged into a serious depression such that she refused to move even the healthy part of her body. Mrs. A. was no longer able to return to her house alone or with a caregiver. She was forced to enter into a nursing home, without even being able to pass by into her house, to collect few objects representing the dearest affections to take with her or saying goodbye from all that she would have left behind her or to choose to give away to relatives or friends.

The anger and the distress, as well as the important depression, made it very difficult to deal with her and any approach of the nursing staff was helpless. During the nights, in a state of anxiety, she constantly rang at the bell to ask for the nurses' help. The situation had become unsustainable for everyone, until an occupational therapist was asked to try to find a solution, building a therapeutic alliance to improve the staff working time and quality.

After an initial approach and assessment, the occupational therapist understood that the goal of "improving wheelchair movements to be more independent within the structure, through increasing motor's coordination and functions," was not significant for Mrs. A. whom she considered the hemiplegic limb useless and dead, and herself so miserable, and physically weakened, that it was not worth the effort to improve her situation. She was so mad that she refused any proposal and was not interested in meeting other residents or entering the dining room to eat meals together. She had close in herself, she self-detained in her room, but at the same time she continuously asked for a massive intervention by the treating staff to reduce her anxiety or to satisfy every movement or need. First, it was necessary to go through the bereavement that she would not be able to return at home anymore and that she would not find anymore the autonomous life of which she was proud in her 84 years of life. The challenge for the therapist was to find, in a relationship of trust, the "access way" to reach Mrs. A. at her core, giving her back the volition to act and to start to consider a new dual therapeutic relationship. The woman had to be able to make a change of perspective and no longer think that the care should only be given "for" her, but that it was still possible to work "with" her. Starting from her life stories (teacher of primary school and passionate travelers to discover the most beautiful areas of Switzerland), with a great cognitive resource (which the stroke did not affect), it had been possible to enter into a relationship through a work of reminiscence.

Initially the occupational therapist was coming regularly to talk to her, showing her a calendar where there were several photos of the most famous places in Switzerland. Mrs A. refused to talk and she got angry: she didn't even want to look or turn the pages with her hand (she was right-handed, her vascular accident affected the left side, the right limb had no difficulties). However, she accepted the presence of the therapist, her speaking, turning the pages of the calendar under her eyes, telling her of curiosities or episodes that occurred in certain cities. During the following sessions, the therapist had noticed that the woman's eyes had remained a few seconds longer on a picture and the inspiration of memory had prevailed over the closure and the anger that characterized her. If at the beginning was the occupational therapist to turn the pages, because Mrs. A. refused to collaborate, once re-motivated and aroused her interest, the woman had begun to accept to turn alone the pages of the book and then to tell the anecdotes lived with her students.

Seeing that the stories became increasingly rich and interesting, the therapist offered her to transcribe the stories and create a small album, a personal diary. Mrs. A. dictated small anecdotes about the places she visited, and the therapist took notes, which she then typed on the PC and, printed on paper. After that the occupational therapist submitted these pages to Mrs. A. that has the task to rereading and correcting them. The lady had rediscovered the ancient pleasure of revising a basic duty of a teacher, and this encouraged her to want to meet the therapist more and more often and enter into the subject and the therapy. With patience and pleasure she adjusted the pages and proposed changes to the text, becoming proactive and adding missing parts and anecdotes that are more and more fun and personal. Slowly, she could begin to talk about her memories and her emotions. And the well-being perceived in re-experiencing memories reassured her and accompanied her for the rest of the day. She was now less bored, less distressed, less angry, and slowly even during the night the doorbell did not ring continuously. Suddenly she began to want to draw and, since the occupational therapist could only come twice a week, they organized themselves so that the lady, in the remaining days, could draw and write independently, thoughts, memories, anecdotes to be reviewed, and shared with the therapist during the scheduled sessions. The anger faded away and left room for deeper feelings and desires to meet, both with the care staff and with other residents. Only at that point Mrs. A. begin to desire to leave the room and to go down to the living room to meet "the people of the house." It was now possible to work on one of the first goals: improving the independently mobility with the wheelchair within the structure, to reach the different spaces and activities to participate actively at the life of the elderly home.

As we can see, the first goal set in occupational therapy had not been to learn the use of a new wheelchair and to train some tips to move in the elderly's residence, but it was to agree on the placement of a table in her room, becoming the "teacher's desk," where she was able to revive and to rediscover her role and the occupation that was part of her life stories. Once the table was accepted, it was essential to find the element, which allowed to enter in an "occupational dialogue." The room was so small that allow the bed and the bedside table. There was only one choice: either the desk or the sofa. The occupational therapist had negotiated for the desk and folding chairs to accommodate any guests. The ever-present anger caused her to reject any proposal, until her eyes lingered on those images that had aroused new interest and passion.

Discovering a new pleasure in going to the living room or dining room and meeting the peers who lived in the residence, had brought out new interests to which she had never paid attention before. Once, while carefully combing her hair in front of the mirror in the bath, before joining the others in the salon, she asked the therapist to give her a lip-gloss that a nursing assistant had given her. It was amazing to observe how she put the lip-gloss by herself, perfectly integrating the hemiplegic limb and above all to note the satisfaction and the pleasure of taking care of herself again. After a long time of suffering, Mrs. A. could now look herself again in the mirror.

When the anger had finally disappeared, she could also regain possession of that faith and the spiritual dimension that had sustained her throughout her life, but that after the intervention she could not consider, because she was completely blocked and devastated by what had happened to her.

Spirituality had once again become important and significant for her: once the priest had not been able to celebrate Mass because he was stuck in the snow, she began to recite the rosary in the Church, calming the agitation of the presents and actively involving them in the prayer.

This discovering of herself in all her psycho-physical and spiritual dimensions allowed Mrs. A. to live serenely and peacefully the last months of her life, before dying from a complication due to a generalized infection.

This clinical case shows us how sometimes a long journey of patience and perseverance is needed before finding that coupling element that becomes a turning point that suddenly bears fruit at all levels. The nursing staff could then finally get in touch with her because, less angry, she had opened the communication, and could express her best. The intervention of the occupational therapist had allowed to move the personal dynamics and find a way of communication through looking at the pictures, the flourishing of memories and emotions in her mind, to find again the pleasure of the written, the drawing, the correcting, to re-appreciate the encounter of the other, and finally to rediscover their spiritual expression.

The example of Mrs. A. allows us to understand more about how it is a priority to find the well-being and to increase the quality and dignity of life by alleviating the *psycho-affective suffering* caused by fear, anxiety, and then facing *physical suffering* (due to paralysis, joint and movement limitations), *moral suffering* (due to the fact that it is no longer able to return home and fulfill her roles), and *spiritual suffering* (not being able to access the life force that had animated her life until then).

7.4   The Living Will and the Advance Care Planning: Focus on Italy

Finally, at the end of the last legislature in Italy the law "provisions for informed consent and advance directives" was approved (law 2019, 22nd December 2017, published on the official journal on 16th January 2018 and entered into force the following 31st January).

Its development was long, troubled, and anomalous considering that the first proposals for a law on living will dates back to the 80s, and few years are passed since the 9th February 2009, the day in which Eluana Englaro, a young woman that was in persistent vegetative state for 17 years died after a long battle[2] carried out by his father and legal guardian and after the sentence of the Suprema Corte di

---

[2] Made of appeals the Corte di Cassazione (high court of appeal) and to the European Court of Human Rights, appeals to the tutelary judge, criminal reports, assignment conflicts presented by the parliament against the constitutional court, appeals to the administrative justice and to the ministerial guideline (see as reference [26]).

Cassazione[3] (high court of appeal) that, for the first time in our country, authorized the doctors to stop artificial hydration and alimentation, respecting the will expressed in advance by the person. This delay denotes that in Italy the bioethical debate is harsh and that exists a distance between the ones who defends the sacrality (and inviolability) of life and the ones who favors its quality [27]. For example, in France the regulation on living will dates back to the *loi* 370 of 22nd April 2005, and it was regulated even before in Belgium with the Act On Patient's Rights of 22nd August 2002. Although the Oviedo Convention, at the article 9 asks the doctor to consider[4] the will expressed in advance by the person if he cannot express it in the present times, the convention was completely ratified only by few European states (in Italy the ratification process begun in 2001 but it is not complete yet because of reasons that everybody knows). Furthermore, also the Italian codex of medical deontology in its version approved by FNMCeo in 1998 encourages the doctors in taking into account the will expressed by the person.

7.4.1 The Italian Law on Provisions for Informed Consent and Advance Directives

The law 219 of 22nd December 2017 was approved at the end of the last legislature with a process that lacked in democracy[5] that accelerated its debate because of electoral reasons and because the center-left coalition who ruled the country decided not to approve the law that granted the citizenship to the person born in Italy from foreign parents.

Art. 1 of the law confirms the personalistic principle laid down in the constitution (as also laid down in the chart of the fundamental right of the European Union) and, with it, medical freedom (art. 32 of the constitution). To exercise this freedom, it is fundamental the right to know and to be informed. This is a wide right that interest also the underaged and the people suffering from mental, cognitive, and intellective

---

[3] High court of appeal, sect 1, 16th October 2007, nr. 21,784. Informed consent, report the supreme judges, is linked to the possibility to choose not only among different care options but also to refuse therapy and to choose to stop it at every time during the life course, even the terminal one. This comply with the personalistic principle that, as said by the court, animates the constitution, since it considers the person itself as something with ethic value that could not be exploited for heteronymic purpose, it conceives the social and solidal actions as a way to improve the person and it speaks about respect of the human being, as individual, in every moment of its life, it considers the integrity of the person and it respects the ethical, religious, cultural, and philosophical beliefs that guide its will.

[4] The expression "to consider" do not imply the fact that the will of the person will be binding, as stated by the explaining report attached to the convention that reports two situations in which the doctor could deviate from the behavior expected: (a) if the will was expressed long time ago; (b) if the state of the art reaches progress that, at the time of the expression of the will, was not envisaged.

[5] With the mechanism of the "kangaroo," an Italian procedural artifact that permitted to condense in blocks more than 6000 amendments presented by the opposition, and, after the discussion of the first and its rejection, all the following blocks were rejected without discussion.

disabilities and remaining the right not to be informed and to empower someone else of to be informed. This freedom is confirmed by the codex of medical deontology (art. 32) and by the Oviedo Convention (art. 10) even if it is not yet completely ratified (the parliament begun the ratification process in 2001). The times and the places dedicated to accrue it not always correspond with the efficiency of the Italian Health System, with its budget and with the rewarding system fastened to the logic of the DRG (diagnosis-related group). It is true that communication is a wonderful time and place for the healing process (art.1 sub 8) in which the autonomies, the responsibilities, and the humanities of the health meet, but at the same time the person needs full respect, and the expression of his will has not to be just a formal-bureaucratic act. Unfortunately, this is what will happen because the new law states that the will has to be expressed in written form, or, when imposed the health conditions of the interested, videotaped (art. 1 sub. 4). This way of acting, associated to the fact that the will expressed in this form exonerate the doctor from any criminal or civil liability (art.1 sub. 6) and from the bond of financial invariance (art. 7) makes the healing process bureaucratic and betrays its purposes and objectives: to build, with human effort and responsibility, a strong and healthy alliance based on mutual knowledge and respect and communicative integrity. The consent is not the collection of a signature on a printed sheet in which the risks will be amplified in order to widen the "protective umbrella" of the legal responsibility; it has to be the conclusion, never hypostatic, of a dynamic and logical process that exploits communication to create a trustee alliance made vital by the gathering (and not the clash) of genuine humanities. A healthy reciprocity that do not end in a signed sheet (collected in the medical record or in the electronic health record) or in a videotaping, but that became history through the communicative process and its gradual and progressive construction of meaning. Speaking about care, communication happens in particular conditions that is a highly asymmetrical relationship, even if doctors usually do not take into account the role difference. The two polarities interested are in irreconcilable and different positions, even antithetical: there is the one who suffers against the one who has to help; the one who knows against the one who knows nothing; the one who has to act against the one who depends on the abilities of the other. As a consequence, what the patience asks to and expects from the doctor is different from what the doctor asks to the patient. The help relationship is based on the impartial openness towards the one who suffers, it is not reciprocal as happens in love relationships, that is, it does not depend (and have not to) on the type of patient and on its personality, census, or race. For this reason, the tasks laid down in the new law have to be contemplated inside (first of all by the doctors) and related to the acts of care. That means that they do not have to be done as a simple bureaucratic activity as has happened in the case of informed consent who was, since today, the collection of a signature on a printed sheet. The communication directed to the creation of the advance directive is a process that needs dedicated places and long times. The new task laid down by the law forecasts a methodical discussion with the patient, as it has to be in all the care relationships, in order to give to him all the information about his clinical conditions, to support him in facing the related stress and to help him in expressing the way in which he wants to deal with pain and death collecting his will.

A prerequisite for this task is the capacity to evaluate the understanding capacities of the patient, his sensitivity and his emotional status and, consequently, the doctor has to be attentive in choosing the right time and place in which give information and collect the will. This process is an active part of the care and it entails commitment and the ability to speak and to be close to the one in pain. Communicative processes are based not only on words, even if they have a fundamental role in transmitting (or not) the semantic content of an information. Words are important but they have to be understandable, concrete, and sober, not banal; they have to be real, to be able to speak to the patient without being in medical technical language. An effective communication requests, before words, empathy and the ability to listen to the other speaker, real communication implies that the speakers have to recognize each other, have to be close and feel close. The doctor has to reach an emotional position based on a delicate and equilibrate mix between distance and compassion that permits empathy, emotional involvement and, at the same time, self-control. In other words, in order to be really and deeply close to the patient and to help him in collecting his final will, the doctor has to be serene and has to mirror the patient; this last has to sense that the doctor could talk about death (this is the matter, alas) without awkwardness. This intimate behavior helps the patient in facing the seriousness of the argument that is directed related to his conditions, in order to carry on a dialogue with himself about his death. All this will happen if ethics do not become a synonym for legality and if the humanities and the responsibilities of the care are protected. To strengthen, even only on the regulatory fields, poorly human relationships improve the yet existing crisis between health and society, invigorating the bureaucratic aspects of the first. In this way, the only task of the medical organizations will be the acquisition/purchasing of the electronic devices intended to videotape the denies of the patients in order to safeguards the professionals. And that was not the aim of that humanization of the healthcare that a lot of people wished for.

The idea laid down in art. 1 sub 5, that artificial alimentation is a therapeutic measure and not a basic physical support could be shared. As a consequence, these treatments are licit only if the patient agrees to them, if they are not therapeutic futility (art. 2 sub 2), if the patient could revoke the consent stopping ongoing medical treatments, if the refusal do not imply abandon, if the patient could receive palliative care (also spiritual and human) that grants him a decent death, and if the patient does not ask illegal health treatments or treatments that go against the deontology and the good practices (art. 1 sub 6). As stated by Pope Francis in the Message to the Pontifical Academy for life on the sixth of November 2017, refusing care "one does will not to cause death: one's inability to impede it is merely accepted," and "not adopting or suspending disproportionate measures means avoiding overzealous treatment." What is needed to be discussed is the idea that the validity of the consensus has to be subjected to the age of consent and to the legal capacity of the person (art. 1 sub 5). Not only because, on international basis, the minors are legally recognized (as stated by UN convention on child's rights) but also because legal capacity is a juridical category that discriminates people (especially the ones who suffer from mental or psychogeriatric illness) and declass them to human beings that cannot exercise the rights and the freedoms innate in every person, making no difference among the various neuro-psychiatric illness and the different stages of the pathologies, strengthening the stigma towards people considered incompetent and incurable. This approach defeats the work carried out for years by the ones who recognize the freedom of the person and digs out outdated interpretations and, in the case of current or advanced informed refusal, custodial care approaches. These people are full-fledged people. There is the need to fight the stigmas and prejudices produced by psychiatric illness, dementia, and *ageism*. Clinical experience illustrates that, very often, a legally incapacitated person is able to make independent moral decisions that need to be respected, provided that the dignity of the person will not be violated. To make the competence, that is an ethic concept, (or the decision-making capacity) banal, and to make it synonym with ability to act or mental competence, that are two not overlapping juridical categories, will encourage the doctor to act in a defensive-bureaucratic way in order to exploit the "protective umbrella" of the civil and criminal irresponsibility [28]. In this way forensic psychiatrist will face overwork because they will be called in the hospital wards in order to evaluate the mental competence of the people that refuse care with the concrete danger that mandatory health treatments become a weapon to standardize inconvenient decisions. Because, usually, it is only in case of refusal that the doctor doubts about the mental competence of the patient, which does not happen when the treatments proposed are welcomed. This legal provision will cause the spread of not virtuosic praxis and danger stereotypes because it cancels the efforts made in the past to educate doctors to consider dementia and neuro-psychiatric pathologies as highly unstable phenotypic character disturbances and mental defect a legal artifact that do not take into account the development of psychic disturbances. The aim is to fight the automatisms that, in the psychogeriatric field, indicate an inadequate professional style or the attempt to trivialize complexity, because every patient has a biographical identity that needs to be protected, respected, and promoted. Art. 3 of the new law takes into account the issue of the minors and the incompetent, illustrating the roles of the parents, the guardian, the curator, and support administrator, although this last had to be more and better delineated. These legal representatives have to pursue the best interest of the person; they have to express his voice without act against him and without give rise to conflicts that might derive from the refusal of medical treatments proposed in the interest of the person, often with the claim of inappropriate therapies. The doctor has to fulfill the interest of the patient and, in case of disagreement, to involve the tutelary judge, is a not convincing nor rational idea. Not only because the time that takes the jurisdiction is not in line with the interest of the patient, but also for the following clear reasons: because jurisdiction is hierarchical and foresees various degrees of judgment; because the tutelary judge, generally, cannot resolve on his own the quarrel between the parts and because this choice will question the role of the doctor in the care relationship. To subordinate doctor's freedom to the jurisdictions means to subordinate scientific knowledge to the laws, even if its independence is awarded by the Constitution; taking into account that the reference only to the good medical practices laid down in art. 1 sub 6 of the new law clashes with the provisions of the Gelli-Bianco law on safeness of care and on professional responsibility.

Art. 4 and 5 of the new law laid down, separately, the right of the person to formalize his advance directives about care options (DAT) and shared care plan.

While sharing this general scheme, there is to worry about some linguistical choices of the legislator and some other questions. First, art. 4 have had to talk about instructions and not about advances directives, then is not persuading the way in which they have to be collected, i.e., as laid down in sub. 6, public act or private agreement and, in the last, they have to be delivered personally to the registry office of the municipality of residence or to the (not better defined) health facilities. The problem lies not in the fact that the DAT have to be expressed in written form, signed and dated, but in the existence of a double procedural course that will favor notaries that, although being technically incompetent, will exercise a hetero-directed external control with the absence of the doctor, both the family doctor or the specialist who is in charge of the care of the person. This is not to transform a personal choice into a clinical choice, but to give to it a clear, accurate, and not questionable content in order to give to it concrete enforceability. Because subsidiarity principle, not only by a technical but also by a human point of view, in this particular moment of the life have to face with responsibility the doubt, held the fear and deal with the stress caused by the unknown.

It is true that, in this document, a person could (not have to) indicate its keeper without bureaucracy, choosing it among his friends or family, but, at the same, worries that, differently from the French Code, there is no clearness on its public role and this could create confusion with others legal representatives, if nominated. It is not clear why, if not nominated, the keeper has to be chosen by the tutelary judge and it could be also the support administrator. The law will be had to encourage the person in always choosing his keeper, being this person not in charge to control the doctors but, above all, being the voice of its beneficiary, knowing his principles, values, identity, and humanity. The function and the importance of the keeper are, in this way, lowered to a subordinate level, underlying that the legal competence (translated in mental capacity in sub. 1 of art. 4) is requested both to the person and to the keeper; and this is an error that, again, discriminates people.

It is not right that the doctor could respect DAT only partially, going completely or partially against them, in accordance with the keeper, if they seem incongruous with the clinical status of the patient or if, when written, there were not therapies able to improve the clinical condition of the patient (art. 4 sub 5). There are instruments able to fight these possibilities, i.e., the updating of the DAT or, as stated before, write the DAT with the help of a doctor, the only one who could explain to the patient in which clinical condition they become effective or the state of the art. To turn to the tutelary judge in the case of clash between the doctor and the keeper shown that the jurisdiction is not the place in which resolve conflicts that pertain to the field of the care. For example, to obtain a second opinion from independent and qualified experts, as happens in other European States, would gave to the law the maturity that is expressed in other articles.

Art. 5 illustrates the shared care plan that is a central theme, as showed by all the international experiences, because of the increase of life expectancy and because of the effect of the epidemiological transaction. It foresee that a person affected by a chronic disease or by a pathology with negative progress (sub 1), after being informed (sub 2), could express his will about the medical treatments to undergo and could give advance directives, included the designation of a keeper (sub 3). They could be periodically updated in relation to the evolution of the disease, if requested by the patient or by his doctor (sub 4). This general scheme could be shared, but it is not clear why there is such a procedural misalignment because, compared to the expression of the will, there is no hetero-directed control apart from a forced call to the jurisdiction in case of a dispute between the doctor and the keeper (sub 5). Furthermore, the function of this last had to be better explained in order to avoid the problems that usually arise in case of uncertainty. Art. 7 laid down a financial invariance clause, revoking the construction of the DAT database, as expressed in the text approved by the commission. This forcing put into risk this freedom, but fortunately, it was corrected with an amendment to the stability law of 2018 who gives two millions of Euros to the health department in order to build the database that had to be ready in June 2018. This did not happened, even if, without this correction, it was not clear how people and professional could use advance directives, unless, in an era of paper dematerialization, the patient had to bring with him a copy of the document, insisting on the fact that doctors, before reanimation, had to search in his pockets for not clearly what.

The approval of the law on living will in Italy was welcomed by a lot of enthusiastic supporters who stated his qualities and underlined the fact that, finally, the country has a law on bio-testament that will avoid situations as the one experienced by Eluana Englaro and Dj Fabo (a young tetraplegic completely blind because of an accident happened in 2014 who was carried in Switzerland by a notorious politician to end his sufferance and was then accused of help in suicide).[6] Fewer people noticed that the law, even having lot of qualities, suffers limits and flaws that needs to be corrected, but, by this point of view, optimisms lack because the database foresee by the stability law of 2018 is not yet into force and the municipality continues to collect living wills in written form without giving to them digital form. Without this last it is really difficult to make concrete the right of a healthy person to express in advance his care options. How it is possible that the new law on informed consent and advance directives, that was object of political fight and not civil attention, could transform itself in concrete (and not bureaucratic) practices and relationships and in adequate times, places, and cultures? This question is not rhetoric. It is really difficult to be optimistic, even because scientific society, with only one exception

---

[6] The Corte D'Assise of Milan asked to the constitutional court to discuss the case because there are gaps in the laws about the constitutional protection of the end of life. The court underlines that the actual laws on end of life do not protect situations that need to be protected and balanced with other constitutional relevant matters. In order to permit to the parliament to act, the court decided to postpone the discussion on the constitutionality of the article 580 of the criminal code to the session that will be hold on 24th September 2019.

(i.e., Associazione Italiana di Psicogeriatria), since now played a passive role, because the good and high principles have to be integrated inside the health and the civil fields improving the professional's way of acting and stopping bureaucratic deviation. In this way humanity could prevail on technicism to create a strong, healthy, and respectful alliance that makes of the care something that is built on human coordinates and not on formal and technical basis.

Without this commitment it is not clear if the new law will be good or bad. I want to believe in it, thinking about the fact that to believe is not a fleeting mood but a virtue that request perseverance, accuracy and, above all, commitment.

Key Message

1. Palliative care is an approach that improves the quality of life and patient and treatment of pain and other problems, physical, psychosocial, and spiritual. The World Health Organization recognizes palliative care among global fundamental strategies for universal health coverage.
2. Since occupational therapy is a rehabilitative health profession that promotes health and quality of life through employment, emerges clearly as such a figure fully belongs to the fundamental ones to reach the goals that palliative care sets for itself.
3. Research has shown that participation in occupations at the end of life is essential for maintaining meaningful relationships, for a sense of effectiveness; they have a strong impact on the person's living environment and an important reflection on everyday life.
4. Palliative care is not only represented by terminal care in people with oncological diseases: even in the geriatric field, palliative care can be a long-term illness intervention, with reality of life that can still be very intense and diversified. However, not all the elderly need palliative care.
5. Although the Oviedo Convention, at the article 9 asks the doctor to consider the will expressed in advance by the person if he cannot express it in the present times, the convention was completely ratified only by few European states (in Italy the ratification process begun in 2001 but it is not complete yet).

References

1. Feifel H, editor. The meaning of death. New York, NY: McGraw-Hill; 1959.
2. Parkes CM. Effects of bereavement on physical and mental health-a study of the medical records of widows. Brit Med J. 1964;2(5404):274–9.
3. WHO definition of palliative care. Available from: www.who.int/cancer/palliative/definition/en.
4. Worldwide Palliative Care Alliance World Health Organization. Global atlas of palliative care at the end of life. 2014.
5. Mingardi B, Monti M, Hartmann E, Castellani L. La terapia occupazionale in hospice: una esperienza preliminare. La Rivista Italiana di Cure Palliative. 2007;1:31–8.

6. Pizzi M. The role of occupational therapy in end of life care. Am J Occup Ther. 2011;65(6):66–75.
7. Pearson EJ, Todd JG, Futcher JM. How can occupational therapists measure outcomes in palliative care? Palliat Med. 2007;21(6):477–85.
8. Russell M, Bahle-Lampe A. The care for the dying: a critical historical analysis of occupational therapy in hospice. Open J Occup Ther [Internet]. 2016;4(2). Available from: https://scholarworks.wmich.edu/ojot/vol4/iss2/12.
9. Costa A, Othero M. Palliative care, terminal illness, and the model of human occupation. Phys Occup Ther Geriatr. 2012;30(4):316–27.
10. Cunningham J. Essere nel fare. Milano: Ed. Franco Angeli; 2006. 45 p
11. Kielhofner G. Model of human occupation: theory and application. 4th ed. Baltimore, MD: Lippincott, Williams & Wilkins; 2008.
12. Hunter EG. Legacy: the occupational transmission of self through actions and artifacts. J Occup Sci. 2008;15(1):48–54.
13. Kaye P. Notes on symptom control in hospice and palliative care. Machiasport, ME: Hospice Education Institute; 2006.
14. Lyons M, Orozovic N, Davis J, Newman J. Doing-being-becoming: occupational experiences of persons with life-threatening illnesses. Am J Occup Ther. 2002;56(3):285–95.
15. Marcil WM. The hospice nurse and occupational therapist: a marriage of expedience. Home Health Care Manag Pract. 2006;19(1):26–30.
16. Saarik J, Hartley J. Living with cancer-related fatigue: developing an effective management programme. Int J Palliat Nurs. 2010;16(1):6–12.
17. Keesing S, Rosenwax L. Establishing a role for occupational therapists in end-of-life care in Western Australia. Aust Occup Ther J. 2013;60(5):370–3.
18. Latini C. La terapia occupazionale nelle cure palliative: quali prospettive in Italia? Giornale Italiano di Terapia Occupazionale GITO. 2013;10(/11):74–80.
19. Park Lala A, Kinsella EA. Phenomenology and the study of human occupation. J Occup Sci. 2011;18(3):195–209.
20. Hammill K, Bye R, Cook C. Workforce profile of Australian occupational therapists working with people who are terminally ill. Aust Occup Ther J. 2017;64(1):58–67.
21. La Cour K, Josephsson S, Luborsky M. Creating connections to life during life-threatening illness: creative activity experienced by elderly people and occupational therapists. Scand J Occup Ther. 2005;12:98–109.
22. La Cour K, Josephsson S, Tishelman C, Nygård L. Experiences of engagement in creative activity at a palliative care facility. Palliat Support Care. 2007;5(3):241–50.
23. Occupational therapy practice framework: domain and process (3rd edition). Am J Occup Ther. 2017;68(Supplement_1):S1.
24. Ardia M, Caiata-Olgiati G. La fragile piuma, Io ergoterapista: corpo, mente, spirito. Ergotherapie. 2007; Bern: ASE.
25. Kübler Ross E. La morte e la vita dopo la morte. Roma: Ed. Mediterranee; 2002.
26. Casini C. Il dibattito sulle dichiarazioni anticipate di trattamento. Valutazioni e prospettive. Medicina e morale. 2010;5(617):62.
27. Fornero G. Bioetica laica e bioetica cattolica. Milano: Ed Mondadori; 2009.
28. Cembrani F, Trabucchi M, Ferrannini L, Agostini C. Capacità ed incapacità al banco di prova della nuova legge sul biotestamento: i tempi della vita nel traffico di un diritto (sempre meno) gentile. Responsabilità medica. 2018;3:1–9.

The Present and the Future of Occupational Therapy

8

Christian Pozzi, Stefano Cavalli, Cristian Leorin, Omar Cauli, and Alessandro Morandi

8.1 Introduction and Background

The title of our chapter leads to consider a time dimension made up of a present and an uncertain future. Commonly, doctors, therapists and other professionals who are engaged in the treatment of frail older people insist in the consideration of the "here and now", the present. In this chapter, we will try to analyse how the occupational therapy may impact on social aspects of the elderly and, vice versa, how social aspects affect occupational therapy, without distinction of disability or pathology, but reflecting on the combination between the present and the future giving rise to an *instant future*. It is not an oxymoron: it is the time in which we are living today. Because among many things that have been vertiginously changed over the years there is also our sense of time and in particular of the future. "The future is not what it used to be" reads a sign on a wall in the middle of Milan. We do not know what it meant to those who made it, but either way, it is absolutely right. The future is almost faster to build than to imagine by now, so much is the speed of change in recent years. This perception varies depending on different stages of people's life.

C. Pozzi (✉) · S. Cavalli
SUPSI - University of Applied Sciences and Arts of Southern Switzerland, Manno, Switzerland
e-mail: Christian.pozzi@supsi.ch; Stefano.cavalli@supsi.ch

C. Leorin
University of Padova, Padova, Italy

Novilunio Association, Padova, Italy

O. Cauli
Department of Nursing, University of Valencia, Valencia, Spain
e-mail: Omar.Cauli@uv.es

A. Morandi
Department of Rehabilitation and Aged Care, Unit of the Ancelle Hospital, Fondazione Teresa Camplani, Cremona, Italy

© Springer Nature Switzerland AG 2020
C. Pozzi et al. (eds.), *Occupational Therapy for Older People*,
https://doi.org/10.1007/978-3-030-35731-3_8

The *instant future* [1] is an absolutely subjective, non-universalistic dimension. Some say, with preoccupation, that we live in an omnivorous present that has devoured both the past and the future. Simply, the boundaries between past, present and future have become much less clear and slide much more easily in the other. The past is now much more present; if only because we have it all available on the web. It is a lot easier than before to access in a few instants to materials and information once difficult and slow to find. As for the future, here we are in that instant future that we have envisioned at the beginning: dynamic, not far, alive in our thoughts. It is the future brought into the world directly from who perform research and projects, invents, tests. It is the future of DNA research, of man on Mars, of new techno-communicational frontiers. It is the future of those looking for a better quality of life through more innovative architectural constructions, interactions between more significant people, truly personalized care. So we will work both in the present and in the future of occupational therapy through a present advanced toward the future trying to give a new boost to building on occupational therapy, to enhance the quality of life, the independence and the autonomy of older people. This push to build is essential to not move away the future from the here and now, rather tie it to the present and to the good practices written in the previous chapters leaving, however, to glimpse other goals to reach.

8.2   The Interaction Between Occupational Therapy and Social Aspect in the Elderly

8.2.1   The Assessment of Social Aspects in Occupational Therapy

Taking into account a therapeutic setting, the first issue of this "sudden future", especially in occupational therapy is to consider social aspects. As a single sentence could not be completely understood when extracted from a wider discussion, in the same way to comprehend an action or occupation is essential to consider the context in which it takes place. To avoid eye contact during the initial interview could be misread as lack of motivation or interest in the therapy, when in some countries and cultures (e.g. the Vietnamese [2]) it is a form of respect. Or, for example, the fact that an old Italian male client has difficulty in choosing what to wear for an evaluation does not necessary mean that he is incapable of make decisions; probably, in the past his wife used to choose his work outfits. The term "social context" concerns the whole situation, the background of the action and the setting in which the action takes place. As it is, it seems to include all the social aspects, but below a distinction among social, personal and cultural contexts will be made, although terms as genre and values are already been used. Avoiding to pay attention to personal, social and cultural media could bring a misunderstanding of evaluations and communications favouring the replacement of a person by dysfunctional cliché. It is obvious that the occupational therapist has to evaluate and take into account all the personal, social and cultural aspects that could help or obstruct the performances carried out during the evaluation period of the therapy. Examples will be provided in clinical practice in order to give the reader a through overview on those fields and on their evaluations.

> **Example 1**
> A 50 years old housewife cooks scrambled eggs for her kids who are returning home from high school, while another 50 years old married woman cooks scrambled eggs for the customers of the cafe shop she owns.

The social role illustrated in the example above is explained in various occupational therapy models and theoretical frameworks. All these models underline the dynamic relationship among human being, environment and occupation. As stated by the World Health Organization (WHO), it is clear that social and cultural background are peripheral to diagnosis and pathology; they are independent but affected by them. It can be affirmed that, in the geriatric field, the occupational therapy "sudden future" requires an appropriate, accurate and evidence-based assessment of:

– *Personal context*: the person's inner environment derived from his/her routine habits, values, beliefs, culture and mood; the person's motor and procedural/cognitive, interpersonal and communication competences enabled during the occupational performance; his/her socioeconomic status; his/her life course.
– *Social context*: the human (role, family) factors that facilitate or hamper the occupational performance of the person.
– *Physical context*: the non-human context (physical spaces, rooms, buildings).
– *Cultural context*: the rules and the values that regulate the society and the community in which the occupational performance takes place.

Here these factors have been separated for pedagogical purposes, but in the daily life they are interconnected and they influence each other in a dynamic way.

8.2.2   Caregiver Adaptation: Promoting Health in Occupational Therapy

An original and obviously interesting theme in the geriatric and psychogeriatric fields, above all for the occupational therapist, is the active involvement of the person with dementia in the various settings that favour the rehabilitation process (see Chaps. 4, 5, and 6 for a detailed discussion of this topic). Thinking in wide terms, in order to give the right importance to social domains it is essential to underline how the rehabilitation process could and has to be shifted into the familiar and social realms of the person (i.e. friends, acquaintances and the wider community). As a consequence, it is essential to involve the caregiver and to promote his/her active role in the rehabilitation process. How to define the term caregiver? It is easy: a domestic caregiver, or domestic assistant, is the unpaid person who helps a non-self-sufficient relative (i.e. for old age or because of having a chronic degenerative disease) because of an emotional bond [3]. Whether full- or part time, the assistance has to fulfill all the needs of the relative assisted. The activities carried out by the caregiver have to comply with the physical (e.g. household chores, administration of drugs and meals), administrative (e.g. collection of retirement benefits or rent) and emotional needs of the assisted, and, in general, with everything that motivates the assisted to be active throughout the day. Furthermore, the caregiver has to supervise the elderly person who could potentially be affected by problems related to the performance in significative activities, or even occupational deprivation in order to avoid harmful and dangerous situation. Depending on the health conditions of the relative assisted, the daily emotional commitment of the caregiver could be so deep that he/she could face psychological problem as anxiety, depression, fear and insomnia [4]. Thanks to his/her knowledge and peculiarities, the occupational therapist has to collect, analyse and comprehend the current, sudden future and future needs and points of view of the caregiver in order to begin a process that leads to a new perception of the assistance thanks to a substantial increase of the sense of competence. The caregiver should not be only an actor in the final stages of the rehabilitation process but should be an actor in each stage of the process (initial assessment, goal setting and planning discharge). As stated by Mosley et al. [5] it is crucial to recognize the actual level of care provided by the caregiver in order to carry out an effective management of the situation. Indeed, in the clinical field it is easy to witness a management only directed to the older person. Rehabilitation processes performed in this way often bring positive outcomes but, in facts, they can be barely generalized. To improve the quality of life of the caregiver, to safeguard his/her job and to prevent an excessive assisting charge it is essential to realize the inclusion of three actors:

- The older person with occupational disabilities;
- The caregiver who is responsible for the assistance;
- The occupational therapist who works inside an interdisciplinary network of professionals.

Didactically speaking, Example 2 shows that the occupational therapist could help the caregiver in order to improve the management of the elderly person with occupational impairment.

It is important [6]:

1. To define the objective and subjective needs of the caregiver and to understand his/her point of view;
2. To define the coping strategies of the caregiver
3. To define the competences that the caregiver perceives to have
4. To agree with the caregiver the target(s) to achieve
5. To involve the caregiver by/in giving recommendations without causing stress

To emphasize point 2, the way in which people cope with stressful situation determines whether or not they avail themselves of healthcare services or whether or not they follow the suggestions of professionals. Coping methods pertain to the person. They could be more or less constant during the life course and it seems that they could compensate stress effects. To avoid that the occupational therapy treatments do not reduce the stress level or do not improve the quality of life of the caregiver, it is important to understand the strategies carried out by the caregiver in the past, in order to explain to him/her how the assistance performed could reciprocate his/her personal coping method (Example 2).

> **Example 2**
> A positive-optimistic coping allows a positive point of view on the therapeutic process. Caregivers endowed with a positive-optimistic coping implement active strategies, such as planning the activities to be done, they have a problem-solving approach and cope with the facts instead of avoiding them.

It is clear that the caregiver, carrying out several activities, both ethical and economical, has a central role in the management of the older person who has occupational disabilities. Nevertheless, caregiving is not recognized as a professional activity by some European states. The number of elderly is increasing and consequently increases the number of people who need home assistance. Several European states grant financial and economic benefits to caregivers as, for examples, tax reductions for the companies who support their caregiver employees, or monthly and annual payments of various amount; or even retirement contributions. In this case, as will be shown in the next part of the chapter, new technologies give social support providing teleworking options. In addition, the older person could receive an allowance to be managed by the familiar or non-familiar caregiver.

To conclude, it is important to underline that, in addition to the family, the social needs of the older person have to be fulfilled by relationships and interactions with other people as friends, neighbours and acquaintances. It is obvious, but still worth mentioning (see Chaps. 2 and 3) that the three actors illustrated above (caregiver, older person and occupational therapist) have to live and interact with other social figures (i.e. friends, acquaintances and healthcare professionals) in an interdisciplinary and gratifying social context.

8.2.3 Loneliness, Boredom and Occupational Therapy

After analysing the several contests in which the actors play a part (in this case the stress is on the older persons, on their family caregiver and their occupational therapy), after analysing the social relationship and focusing on the role of the caregiver, we think it would be interesting to consider the individuality of elderly including feelings, wishes and sufferings. This is important because quality of life and personal wellness do not depend only on their objective conditions but also on their expectation, priority, comparison between their situation and other situations or the social representation of ageing.

The huge variety in older populations can be explained by this reason. As a consequence, it is essential that occupational therapists, in their clinical reasoning, take into account these personal aspects.

In this part of the chapter we are focusing on two common aspects that a lot of people who are hospitalized in different settings may feel: loneliness and boredom.

Loneliness and boredom are words that are often connected to people who are hospitalized, for short or long time. Especially for people who have to stay in the hospital for a long time the boredom, more than the pain or the invasive nursing practices, is very difficult to cope with [7].

> **Example 3**
> Boredom is, as many patients will attest, as close to torture as any Dark Ages tormentor could inflict. The pain of the operations, the stripping away of dignity necessitated by weak to non-existent bathroom functions and a constant fixation over pressure sores does not even come close to matching the horror of a mind able only to feed on itself [8].

The person who writes this word is Jeremy Smith after spending 11 months in a hospital due to injury in spinal cord.

During this period he also had an infection and he had to stay in isolation for about 2 months. As a result, he experienced boredom in a very intimate and fraternal way. He says that many doctors and therapists have been able to be compassionate with his anxiety and his worry about the future, but no one has been able to truly understand his boredom and loneliness. As a matter of fact according to Mr. Smith, doctors and therapists focused on and approached to these symptoms as objective and somehow manageable issues. Actually, he considered them to be obvious, inevitable symptoms. They were the result of an institutionalized and slow routine, always the same. Basically, this routine presented its cost. Mr. Smith said that distractions were few, rare and the available ones quickly lost their appeal. Even receiving visitors had become stressful.

Before taking into account a possible assessment, it is important to define the term boredom. Boredom is a common experience but difficult to understand. It is characterized by a feeling of indifference and passive waiting, in addition to a feeling of apathy that makes the subject distant from everything. The bored and the apathetic ones feel like the time has stopped in an eternal present distinguished by lack of pleasure. At first sight, an overlap of the two phenomena seems possible, but is not real because while the apathetic one finds peace in this lack of pleasure, the bored one is anguished by the need of feel again any sensation. How should it be possible to diagnose this condition widely spread also in our rehabilitation settings? Mr. Smith reports how psychotherapists, doctors and therapists had never noticed his state, and had never simply asked him: "How are you? Are you bored?"

In the phenomenology illustrated by Mr. Smith it is discouraging that the actions recorded as distractions, were, in facts, his significant activities, his personal occupations. Evident occupations: books, bright walls, sheets to be written, letters, photos of relatives and friends. So, not only actions or movements but also cosy, pretty, optimistic spaces: yet, often in hospitals measures intended to improve the quality of the spaces are not adopted; on the contrary the spaces are actively spared.

Talking again about boredom or loneliness, it is appropriate to provide the reader with two evaluation scales widely used in the scientific literature of this field. The Boredom Proness Scale [9] measures the problem with accuracy and effectiveness; regarding loneliness and social isolation the Community Integration Questionnaire [10] identifies the settings that could be improved by the rehabilitation process.

The occupational therapist, being focused on the occupations, has to offer to the hospitalized older person little but precious and essential comfort moments intended to create or recreate a link with the family and the home in order to avoid boredom. For example, (one of the authors of this essay well remembers that Mrs. Julie Cunningham, one of his former teachers, gave her hospitalized mother basil plants) flowers and plants, as far as sentimental, embody care and recall to the hospitalized person the world outside. In this case, the occupational therapist, working inside an inter-professional and multidimensional network, could bring the hospitalized elderly to the garden or to outdoor spaces; here he could offer them board games, drawing and writing materials or origami to be done. In this way boredom has to fight against activities and occupations. As occupational therapists, we have to monitor, in an empathetic but determined way, that the activities illustrated above do not become trivial. If not correctly assessed, or if carried out in an inadequate space or without a team able to give to them the correct meaning, these activities could even become counterproductive or could bring to negative outcomes. The knowledge and the peculiarities of the occupational therapist have to improve the take in charge of the occupational domain in order to reduce the feeling of abandonment, boredom and isolation, as well depicted by Mr. Smith.

8.3   Technology and Older Adults

In this chapter, we will see that the beneficiaries of technology can be categorized into three groups. The first includes older people living at home: technology facilitates independent yet safe living, prevents the need to be under institutional care, reduces depression, increases well-being and quality of life. The second category is health care professionals: effective implementation of assistive technology facilitates better independence and integration of the elderly, it reduces overload of work and resulting burnout, it promotes specific rehabilitation interventions and enlarges the occupational therapists' competences. The third group, the health care system, also benefits from use of technology: it advances care service provision and helps to establish a more organized and effective system (using also artificial intelligence) which satisfies the elderly and motivates health care work force.

The concept of self-care includes the ability to care for oneself and the performance of activities necessary to achieve, maintain or promote optimal health. The effort individuals make towards achieving optimal health depends on individual's capacity and personal characteristics such as coping abilities, skills, social life, personal values and level of literacy. For many older people, independence is the core component to measure the quality of life [11]. The main characteristic of positive ageing is how independent individuals are and how much control they have over their own lives [12]. The goals of an occupational therapist are to maximize empowerment, independence and productivity of individuals and their integration and inclusion in the mainstream of society [13].

In order to keep the quality of care uncompromised, implementation of specific technology is believed to contribute a lot to enhance the self-care ability of elderly and eases the workload of social and health carers [14].

8.3.1 What Is Assistive Technology

Assistive technology (AT) is a term used to describe the products and services which enable individuals' functioning and participation. Also known as "aids and equipment", "medical appliances" or "medical devices", the term AT products refers to devices, equipment, instruments and software used by or for persons with disability. Several articles [15–19] point out that the technologies and services start from the experienced needs of the older adults. If they expect to benefit from the devices or solutions, they are likely to have more positive attitudes, and thereby higher motivation to learn to use the technology in question. When an older adult does not see a need for technology, it is unlikely that she/he will be inclined to use it [18]. However, it is highlighted that the usability of the technology is crucial and solutions that were perceived as complex or difficult to learn were easily abandoned soon, whereas devices that were simple were used more often and even after several months [18–20].

From the quality of life aspects, technology may serve several purposes among older adults. It can satisfy the elderly's wish to maintain independence and autonomy, to have social contacts with family and friends, to ensure security and safety and more importantly to maintain dignity to the end of life. At policy level, the issue is further pushed by the UN Convention on the Rights of People with Disabilities (CRPD) that in various articles refers to the role of technology to support participation, access and equal opportunities. However, according to Greenhalgh et al. [17], many technologies serve the health care or social service providers, but do not actually improve the lived experience of impairment of the older adults [17]. Timing of the implementation of technology is often discussed, pointing out the need for proactive training, education and preparation [17, 18]. This is also relevant not only for the EU, but also internationally. Additional research in the US by Scherer [21–23] indicates a continuum of use and non-use, including partial/reluctant use and avoidance of use, resulting from the confluence of personal, environmental and technology factors. See in Fig. 8.1 the assistive technology assessment process ideal model under the lens of the ICF biopsychosocial model [24] with the role of the different specialists.

In Europe, assistive technology service provision became an important part of each country's healthcare and social support policy. The system and the extent of delivery vary from country to country. In some systems, it includes personalized environmental adaptation such as modifications to bathroom, kitchen and general

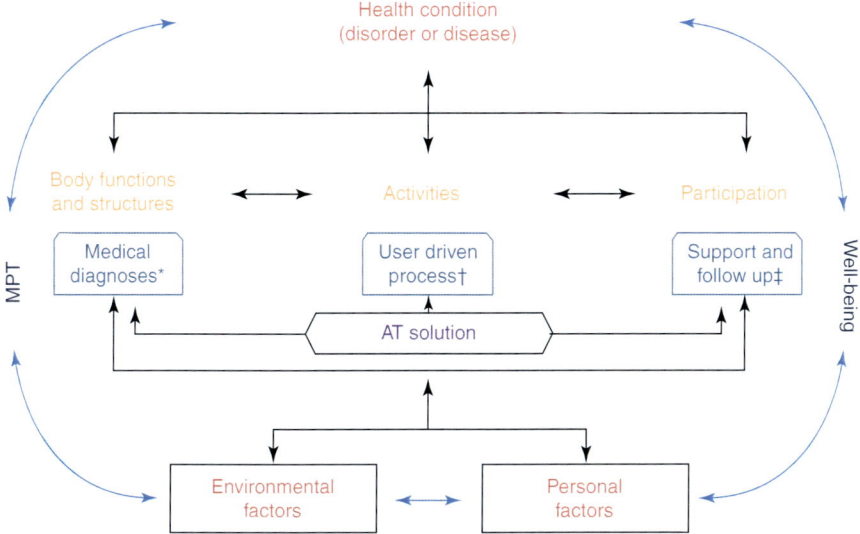

* The physician, the psychologist, the cognitive therapist, the optometrist, the audiologist, the pediatric specialist, the geriatrician.
† The psychotechnologist, the occupational therapist, the architech, the engineer.
‡ The therapist, the special educator, the occupational therapist, the psychologist, the consumer support, speech language pathologist, the physiotherapist.

Fig. 8.1 ATA process ideal model under the lens of the ICF (International Classification of Functioning) biopsychosocial model

areas. While in others, it is limited to products such as prosthetics, wheelchairs, orthotics, hearing aids and foot ware which helps to maintain functional capacity [24]. The variety and availability of technologies and supportive living environments are showing encouraging developments for elderly and people with disabilities to live independently and participate in daily activities [25].

8.3.2   The Classification of the Information and Communication Technologies

Information and communication technologies (ICT) are believed to fill the gap in demand for caring professions without compromising the quality of care. The contribution of technology to elderly care in institutions and at home is under continuous research and development. There are many large European projects about facilitating independent living at home (i.e.: Accompany, Beyond Silos, Perssilaa, Inca, Fate, Carer+, I-Support, Robot-Era, Silver, etc). Currently, assistive technology products such as safety alarms, smart sensors and remotely monitored device are being developed, installed and investigated among other things with the aim of creating different kinds of independent living services to overcome barriers to independence. These services have been defined as "any product, application or service

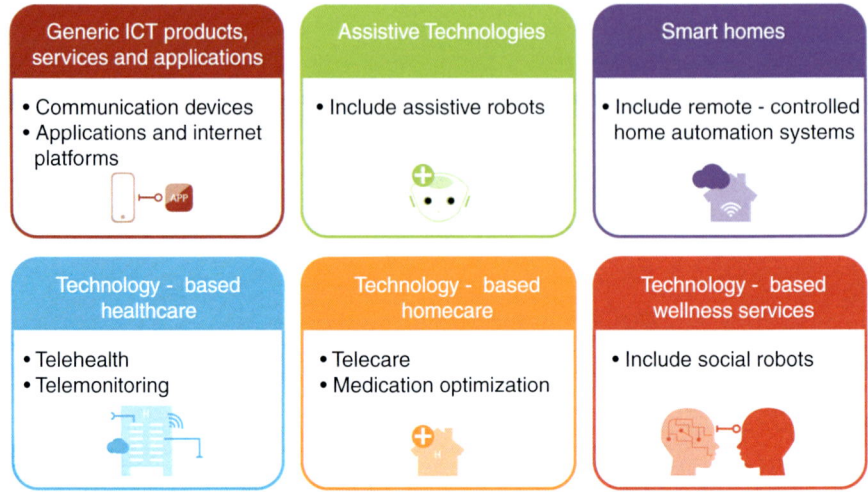

Fig. 8.2 Classification of technology-based services for independent living

that enables people, whose independence in daily life is challenged, to lead a more independent and participatory life" [26].

In specific, as showed in Fig. 8.2, there are many applications and different tools used by elderly people and occupational therapists to maintain independence at home and to be part of the society, most of them with artificial intelligence that positively enlarges the outcomes.

- *Generic information and communication technology products, services and applications.* ICT products, services and applications available in the market and developed for everybody, that play a relevant role as a technology service for the independence of older adults at home. These services include mostly communication devices such as mobile phones and applications on Internet. They can be accessed remotely from the older and disabled people's homes which allow them to engage in a range of activities: e.g. social, working, learning or entertainment activities. For example, teleworking services, information and training platforms, social networking technologies and online services such as those offering tele-shopping or tele-banking.
- *Assistive technologies*, as discussed above, refer to devices and equipment that compensate for sensory, physical/mobility and cognitive impairments. They include voice recognition software, text telephones, accessible keyboards, speech recognition software [27], intelligent electric magnifiers and reading lenses and other assistive devices to drive a car or to do sports [19, 28, 29].
- These technologies also include *assistive robots,* defined as those that help older people with physical disabilities to carry out daily life activities or to recover or maintain some capacity. There are prosthetic robots that replace lost or damaged parts of the body; or mobility aids, i.e. non-prosthetic technology which replace

or extend the functionality of a leg or an arm; robots for training and rehabilitation to be used for individual training, exercises and rehabilitation; and finally robots that carry out logistic and cleaning tasks, which can be used for personal care [30].

- *Smart homes* refer to different ICTs integrated in older people's houses to help them to perform everyday life activities independently. They include remote-controlled home automation systems, which have various sensors for doors and gates, microwaves or normal stoves, security devices, lighting and an on/off switch for various appliances and home entertainment [31]. They can also include generic ICT applications such as online services offering tele-shopping or tele-banking [29]. Smart homes are composed of sensors, actuators, controllers, a central unit, networks and an interface [31]. The ICT components are programmed to react and communicate with each other through a local network, and with the surroundings via the Internet, ordinary fixed telephones or mobile phones.

- *Technology-based healthcare.* The following healthcare technologies can help to prevent, early detect, cure and manage chronic conditions;
  - *Telemedicine* is defined by the WHO as "the delivery of healthcare services, where distance is a critical factor, by all healthcare professionals using information and communication technologies for the exchange of valid information for diagnosis, treatment and prevention of disease and injuries, research and evaluation, and for the continuing education of healthcare providers, all in the interests of advancing the health of individuals and their communities" (2009). Telemedicine involves secure transmission of medical data and information, such as biological/physiological measurements, alerts, images, audio, video or any other type of data needed for prevention, diagnosis, treatment and follow-up monitoring of patients [13].
  - *Telehealth* or disease management applications deliver services from a healthcare provider to a citizen, from one health professional to another, or between citizens and family members [32]. Telemedicine and telehealth are similar and, in many documents, appear as the same concept, but the former refers to service delivery by physicians only, and the latter to services provided by health professionals in general, including nurses, occupational therapists, pharmacists and others (WHO 2009). Home telehealth refers to a range of support, typically including not just clinical (medical) monitoring and intervention, but also a broader range of homecare support that more traditionally falls within the scope of social/homecare services [33].

- *Technology-based home care* refers to the use of ICTs to monitor well-being and to provide a secure home environment. They include:
  - *Telecare and telemonitoring*: this refers to the provision of social care from a distance using telecommunications [34]. The last generation telecare (after the emergency alarms and environment sensors) collects everyday activity data automatically through various sensors such as front door open/closed detectors, fridge open/closed detectors, pressure mats, bed/chair occupancy

and electrical usage sensors. This data is presented to care personnel or family carers to monitor well-being and assess the need for help and support. Several technologies remotely manage and monitor a range of health conditions and collect/send vital signs to a monitoring station for interpretation. A home unit measures and monitors temperature, blood pressure and other vital signs for clinical review at a remote location (for example, a hospital) using phone lines or wireless technology (WHO, 2009).

– *Medication management* refers to a wide variety of technologies designed to help manage medication information, dispensing, adherence and tracking. Technologies range from fully integrated devices that use ICTs to inform and remind stakeholders at multiple decision and action points throughout the patient care process to the simpler, standalone devices with more limited functionality.

• *Technology-based wellness services* deliver services for healthier lifestyles to older and disabled people at home. They include mainly cognitive fitness and assessment technologies, which consist of thinking and cognitively challenging games to maintain or improve cognitive health. Many cognitive fitness technologies are computer or Internet based, and they include an assessment and tracking component. They can also include social robots whose tasks are to maintain some form of interaction, and to engage older adults in natural social exchanges [35]. They give a sense of social presence in an interaction and the capacity for touch and physical interaction [36].

The occupational therapists can help in overcoming barriers to assistive technology use and acceptance by providing information about the previously described areas as well as properly matching assistive devices to a person's needs. The rehabilitation specialist can also aid in overcoming barriers by adequately training a person with the assistive technology device and providing follow-up services to ensure comfort, satisfaction, safety and continued use of the device.

8.3.3 Barriers and Acceptance of Technology in the Elderly

Despite these advances across Europe and internationally, the implementation of technology-based services for independent living is still slow in the Member States mainly due to the following challenges [37]:

• Older people may not have the required digital skills. Equipment, interfaces and services designed to promote healthy and active ageing are not tailored to the functional limitations of older people [19].
• There is still a lack of information and robust studies on the effectiveness and efficiency of these technologies, and this creates a barrier to public and private investment to implement solutions on a wider scale. For example, there is scepti-

cism regarding the ability of technology-based solutions to produce tangible benefits, and there are some areas that have failed to demonstrate the effectiveness of these solutions, despite their innovative potential to increase the health and well-being of older people and their careers.

- There is a lack of understanding of how and where technology-based solutions can benefit long-term care structures and interfaces, particularly with respect to health and social care delivery and integration, and the links between formal and informal care.
- There is little knowledge of the steps that must be taken to scale up technology-based services for independent living for older people [38]. Moreover, there is a lack of efficient business models that could show governments how much the services would cost.
- Transferability of good practice may depend on several variables, such as the national or local characteristics, cultures or habits and the surrounding health and welfare system or the existing support services [37].

Policy could boost the introduction of effective solutions for independent living and provide solutions for the above challenges. Besides providing funding to create, develop and innovate technology-based services for older adults and carers through R&D and innovation programmes (e.g. Horizon 2020 Programmes and Active Assisted Living Joint Programming), one of the main strategies European policy could follow is to promote the exchange of good practices, the collection of evidence and the transferability of optimal solutions to other localities, regions and countries, to encourage the use of existing effective solutions in the EU (i.e.: see EU projects SCIROCCO, SUSTAIN, INTEGRATE).

Technology is not always deployed or researched in a fully consumer-focused way. Many of the studies investigating the use of technology for improving ADL and quality of life show a lack of rationale for choice of technology, little involvement of older people in technology selection, lack of clarity regarding the goals of older people and a lack of tailored approaches [39, 40]. If the end users of assistive technology are not empowered to co-produce and collaborate on the development of AT, a critical opportunity for appropriate co-design is lost. For example, the emerging concerns that surveillance and monitoring technologies may, in fact, be experienced as a form of restraint, show the need for an ethical framework in their application [19, 41]. More research on the social consequences of assistive technologies is also needed, since overcoming these social barriers may depend on their success. Compared to traditional assistive devices, the use of mainstream technology (e.g. smartphones, tablets) has shown more acceptance and increased perception of independence in social contexts, also relevant to issues of Universal Design [42, 43].

The role of an occupational therapist, updated about new technologies and rehabilitation opportunities connected to AT and artificial intelligence, is to maximize empowerment, independence and productivity of individuals and their integration and inclusion in the society.

8.4   Evidence-Based Practice in Occupational Therapy: The Need for Randomized Clinical Trials (RCTs) and Other Research Studies

Research studies designed to demonstrate the efficacy and effectiveness of occupational therapy interventions provide scientific evidence for their benefits and in so, often justify their use. These studies also help to refine and improve the interventions already employed and provide knowledge of their mechanisms of action. They specify the patients in which they are effective, how long the treatments must be applied for, and define the desired outcomes and circumstances for the therapy, as well as any precautions, limitations or alternatives to the treatment. However, to meet all these challenges, occupational therapy researchers must increase the rigour of their research.

From the first randomized controlled trial (RCT), published in 1948 [44], to the current era of "evidence-based medicine", the design of clinical trials and the tools available for analysing the data have become increasingly sophisticated. Nonetheless, more controlled trials of different interventions, especially RCTs, are still needed in order to recommend or implement interventions on large scales. However, we must remember that properly designed RCTs rely on the existence of prior observational studies which investigate treatment outcomes; this is particularly the case in large, heterogeneous populations of patients with complex, chronic diseases [45].

The occupational therapy field has made major strides towards increasing the number of published controlled trials. In the Cochrane Library of clinical trials alone, 171 registered clinical trials appeared in which the words "occupational therapy" and "older" appeared in the Abstract, while 44 contained the words "occupational therapy" and "geriatric" (at the time of writing on 30 January 2019). Moreover, because occupational therapy is broad, it draws evidence from many fields. For instance, searching for RCTs containing the words "work rehabilitation" retrieved thousands of trials, all largely within the scope of the practice of occupational therapy.

Trials of physical agents and interventions in physical medicine and rehabilitation can also be relevant to occupational therapy. For instance, psychological, behavioural, counselling, exercise and educational interventions often involve strategies or methods that are used in occupational therapy, even though they are not usually indexed under this term. Moreover, it is easy to locate thousands of other RCTs relevant to occupational therapy with minimal effort. In the future, these publishing and strategical issues must be clearly defined to facilitate and rationalize both keyword searches and for the assessment of optimal keywords for use in new scientific reports on clinical trials involving aspects related to occupational therapy.

8.4.1   Barriers to RCTs in Occupational Therapy

Despite recent progress, when looking for studies that directly support specific clinical practices, it is common knowledge that one is likely to encounter a dearth of strong scientific evidence. There are many barriers to the conduct of RCTs in occupational therapy. Most of these are familiar, if not sometimes misunderstood, as explained in more detail below.

As in other health-sciences disciplines, which provide non-pharmacological interventions, performing RCTs in the field of occupational therapy entails ethical difficulties, because one cannot prevent patients from receiving a treatment that is likely to help them. Moreover, clinical trials must be conducted in the highly ethical context of good clinical practice.

Even when ethical, RCTs are often infeasible because of practical constraints in the local practice setting, a lack of training among occupational therapists in the required scientific methodology, and, above all, a lack of funding. Although inexpensive or cheap RCTs are possible and should be encouraged [46–48], they are typically more expensive than the qualitative, observational or case-series studies that occupational therapy faculty and graduate students so often carry out with limited or no external funding at all. A case of almost inexpensive trial is based on alternating intervention approaches that work especially well when the intervention treatment is easy to switch, and the studies can be inexpensive when the outcomes are electronically recorded or otherwise easy to obtain.

In general, conducting a RCT (or any other type of controlled trial) typically requires substantial developmental work to create and refine a protocol for a well-defined and specific intervention. Unless the "experimental" intervention is seen as likely to be superior to the standard-of-care treatment, there is usually insufficient justification for the trial.

8.4.2   Specific Issues Related to RCTs in the Field of Occupational Therapy

Clinical trials of occupational therapy interventions present particular challenges. One of these is blinding the research participants to their treatment allocation group. Blinding is necessary to reduce measurement bias as well as the bias inherent to the experimenter. The use of an appropriate control group is also a related concern. In drug trials, the use of placebo controls and participant blinding is relatively easy, but this task is more difficult—and is even sometimes impossible—in non-pharmacological and behavioural interventions including occupational therapy. This is because these interventions usually require directly working through the actions, motivations and experiences of the patient.

Nonetheless, the following procedures may be useful to minimize the biases associated with RCTs in occupational therapy studies:

- The professionals or research assistants measuring the patients' baselines and outcomes should almost always be blinded to the patient allocation.
- Researchers should avoid conveying their expectations for the potential results to the study participants; the principal investigator and staff involved in studies must always keep in mind that unbiased, balanced estimates are the true aim of the work.

- Subjective reports (e.g. client satisfaction or quality of life) are particularly subject to social desirability and other biases [49]. Therefore, it is important to carefully assess the procedures to be used and to ask maximally unbiased questions (e.g. "Are you satisfied or dissatisfied?" rather than "How satisfied are you?").
- Standardized questionnaires with an established reliability and validity must be employed. It is important to remember that questionnaires and scales must be validated for use in the primary language of the patients in which they are applied. If the appropriate scales are not available in the required language, then they should be translated and validated before their use.
- Researchers should implement outcomes such as measures of activity, performance, occupational patterns and time used which are potentially objective, depending on the degree of inter-operator reliability and the procedures used to minimize bias.
- The control group should be the waiting list group, which means that all participants will receive the same intervention, directly or after a while. This enlarges the motivation for participation and deals with ethical dilemmas because in this case the intervention is not kept back for the participants of the control group.

Individual RCTs and systematic-reviews and meta-analyses of RCTs should control for the risk of bias in randomized and placebo-controlled studies according to the guidelines set out in the Cochrane Review guidelines [50] summarized in Table 8.1.

Other methodologies have been normalized for quantitative studies—not only experimental studies such as RCTs, but also for observational studies. An example is the criteria rated by the critical appraisal tool proposed by the Joanna Briggs Institute [51, 52] for studies performed with quantitative methodologies (Table 8.2). This critical appraisal checklist should be considered when designing experimental and observational studies or when performing critical literature reviews and considers the following ten items:

It is crucial for real-word research studies to develop uniform, objective interventions. Although these procedures may increase the cost of clinical trials, other strategies can be used to reduce these costs. For instance, if one studies interventions and outcomes with a high effect size, statistical significance can be reached with small or moderate-sized samples. This means that while designing RCTs, it is crucial to calculate the adequate sample size required to be able to detect a significant effect should the interventions tested indeed have any beneficial effects in the study sample in question.

Table 8.1 Common bias in RCTs

Source of bias	Type of bias
Random sequence generation	Selection bias
Allocation concealment	Selection bias
Blinding of participants and personnel	Performance bias
Blinding of outcome assessment	Detection bias
Incomplete outcome data	Attrition bias
Selective reporting	Reporting bias

Table 8.2 Critical appraisal tool

1	Was the sample representative, as judged by the specific population characteristics such as age, sex and other influential factors?
2	Were the study participants recruited using appropriate sampling methods without bias and inclusive of all possible groups?
3	Was the sample size adequate, and was it supported by a sample size calculation which included subgroup sizes?
4	Were study participants and settings described in detail to facilitate clear comparisons with other data?
5	Was the data analysis conducted with enough coverage of the identified sample and an adequate description of the non-participants?
6	Were objective, standard criteria for the measurements used?
7	Were the methods of measurement reliable and explicitly described?
8	Was there an appropriate statistical analysis?
9	Were all important confounding factors, subgroups or differences identified and accounted for?
10	Were subpopulations identified using objective criteria?

8.4.3 Recommendations

The criteria for necessary and optimal research completely depend on the status of prior research on the topic and on the current barriers to progress. Researchers can and should alter their research objectives and research design to fit the problem they are addressing. Study objectives are still classified as initial, exploratory, confirmatory or use in practice, which correspond to Phases I, II, III, and IV [53]. However, a classification system based on the study objectives might be preferable to these general phases because study objectives can be specified in greater detail.

Promising intervention strategies need to be identified, explored and developed in single-subject design studies or in Phase I research. Any promising interventions from Phase I trials should then be tested in small, exploratory controlled studies (Phase II trials). These small controlled trials can advance knowledge in numerous areas of occupational therapy interventions. After testing in a small controlled trial(s), researchers will be able to design a conclusive or definitive Phase III trial. Basic research and studies of occupational therapy in practice (analogous to Phase IV trials in the drug research field) will also be needed to maintain implementation over time.

Occupational therapy could greatly benefit from a more systematic approach to study development and interventions strategies. However prior to design a clinical or community RCT, a preparatory research (such as pilot studies) is necessary in order to be successful, and often, small trials—Phase II RCT—must be carried out before a large more conclusive trial can be planned. It is import to underlie that in order to build good scientific evidence it is necessary to pass through the different phases of study development. It is important to avoid considering that occupational therapy research should generally be expected to jump directly from preliminary (or theoretical) findings to definitive conclusions via a single "large" RCT.

The development of interventions should be referred to internationally accepted standards regarding methodological rigour and scientific evidence levels [54, 55]. Observational studies such as cross-sectional studies, case-control or cohort studies employ matching or correlational control procedures usually involve many more confounding factors than RCTs and so, the accompanying methodologies to control for selection biases and variations in patient severity are also complex as mentioned above [56, 57]. Nevertheless, it is true that strong, quasi-experimental research designs can likely provide more evidence of effectiveness if these technical requirements are met [58, 59].

Quasi-experimental research shares similarities with traditional experimental designs or RCTs, but specifically lacks the element of random assignment to treatment or control groups. Instead, these designs typically allow researchers to control assignment to the treatment conditions based on some criterion other than random assignment (e.g. an eligibility cut-off point) [59]. In some cases, the researcher may even have control over treatment assignment. Quasi-experiments are subject to concerns about internal validity because the treatment and control groups may not be comparable at the baseline.

With random-assignment quasi-experimental studies, the participants have the same chance of being assigned to the intervention group or the comparison group. As a result, differences between groups, both in terms of observed and unobserved characteristics, are due to chance rather than a systematic factor related to treatment (e.g. illness severity). However, randomisation itself does not guarantee that groups will be equivalent at baseline; while any changes in the patient characteristics detected post-intervention are likely attributable to the intervention, in quasi-experimental studies, it may not be possible to convincingly demonstrate a causal link between the treatment condition and observed outcomes. This is particularly true if there are confounding variables that cannot be controlled or accounted for.

Controlled trials provide a path and an incentive for the development and testing of explicit new interventions, even if they are distinctly different from current practices. In addition, occupational therapy research differs substantially from the study of drugs. It is not hard to argue that RCTs have a more limited application in the study of occupational therapy than they do for drugs. Thus, single-subject design studies may be the design of choice for clarifying the apparent immediate effects on individuals (if not the average long-term benefits to populations) for many occupational therapy interventions (e.g. assistive technology).

However, interventions are best developed and tested in a theoretical framework so that the research results strengthen or modify the theory and might guide future work and generalizations when translated to clinical or community practice. In addition, a basic research into biological processes already provides such a basis for drug studies, but to achieve the same for occupational therapy and behavioural interventions, these fields will have to develop their own theories, incorporating biological knowledge as part of a wider psychosocial whole [60].

This an exciting time in occupational therapy research, a time which has great potential to enhance existing occupational therapy interventions and for the development of distinctly new ones. This can be achieved by testing and demonstrating their effectiveness through experimental studies (RCTs being the best option) for a variety of patient types, settings and desired outcomes. At the same time, occupational therapy research can also contribute to multidisciplinary research and lead to the implementation of practices such on Alzheimer's diseases patients and their caregivers [61–64] that routinely engender greater and more sustained improvements in the lives of individuals.

Key Messages

1. The present and the future are two concepts with a rapid evolution and relationship, especially when considered in the care of elderly people.
2. There is an emerging need around Europe to understand how to approach the ageing population in different cultures.
3. Loneliness and boredom are two conditions often under-evaluated by occupational therapists, which require a specific approach to improve elderly people quality of life in different settings.
4. Technology and assistive technology might represent a venue to improve the occupational therapy management of elderly people. However, it is crucial to understand how to overcome the current cultural barriers and how to provide changes in the technology application for the current and future ageing population.
5. The continuous evaluation of occupational therapy interventions in clinical trials is key to support and provide the scientific evidence for the best approach to elderly people.

References

1. Bolelli F. Come Ibra, Kobe, Bruce Lee. Lo sport e la costruzione del carattere. ADD Editore: Torino; 2018. 125 p.
2. Minarik PA, Lipson JG. Culture and nursing care: a pocket guide. 1st ed. San Francisco: Univ of California San Francisco; 1996.
3. Barnes M. Storie di caregiver. Il senso della cura. Trento: Erickson; 2010; 240 p.
4. Grant JS, Bartolucci AA, Elliot TR, Giger JN. Sociodemographic, physical, and psychosocial characteristics of depressed and non-depressed family caregivers of stroke survivors. Brain Inj. 2000;14(12):1089–100.
5. Mosley PE, Moodie R, Dissanayaka N. Caregiver burden in Parkinson disease: a critical review of recent literature. J Geriatr Psychiatry Neurol. 2017;30(5):235–52.
6. Graff M, Melick MV, Thijssen M, Verstraten P, Zajec J, Fabbo A. Curare la demenza a domicilio. Indicazioni di terapia occupazionale per anziani e caregivers. 1st ed. Milan: Franco Angeli; 2015. 322 p.
7. Martin M. Boredom as an important area of inquiry for occupational therapists. Br J Occup Ther. 2009;72(1):40–2.
8. Smith J. It was only a tiny garden, but it helped me smile again. 2016 gennaio 16 [citato 2019 marzo 20]. https://www.telegraph.co.uk/news/telegraphchristmasappeal/12099804/It-was-only-a-tiny-garden-but-it-helped-me-smile-again.html.

9. Vodanovich SJ. Psychometric measures of boredom: a review of the literature. J Psychol. 2003;137(6):569–95.
10. Salter K, Foley N, Jutai J, Bayley M, Teasell R. Assessment of community integration following traumatic brain injury. Brain Inj. 2008;22(11):820–35.
11. Demiris G, Hensel BK. Technologies for an aging society: a systematic review of "smart home" applications. Yearb Med Inform. 2008;17(1):33–40.
12. Brownie S, Horstmanshof L. Creating the conditions for self-fulfilment for aged care residents. Nurs Ethics. 2012;19(6):777–86.
13. Cason J. Telehealth: a rapidly developing service delivery model for occupational therapy. Int J Telerehabil. 2014;6(1):29–35.
14. Kachouie R, Sedighadeli S, Khosla R, Chu M-T. Socially assistive robots in elderly care: a mixed-method systematic literature review. Int J Hum Comput Interact. 2014;30(5):369–93.
15. Eisma R, Dickinson A, Goodman J, Syme A, Tiwari L, Newell AF. Early user involvement in the development of information technology-related products for older people. Univers Access Inf Soc. 2004;3(2):131–40.
16. Orpwood R. Involving people with dementia in the design process: examples of iterative design. In: Dementia, design and technology. London: IOS Press; 2009. p. 79–95.
17. Greenhalgh T, Wherton J, Sugarhood P, Hinder S, Procter R, Stones R. What matters to older people with assisted living needs? A phenomenological analysis of the use and non-use of telehealth and telecare. Soc Sci Med. 2013;93:86–94.
18. Peek STM, Wouters EJM, van Hoof J, Luijkx KG, Boeije HR, Vrijhoef HJM. Factors influencing acceptance of technology for aging in place: a systematic review. Int J Med Inf. 2014;83(4):235–48.
19. Leorin C, Stella E, Nugent C, Cleland I, Paggetti C. The value of including people with dementia in the co-design of personalized eHealth technologies. Dement Geriatr Cogn Disord. 2019;47(3):164–75.
20. Cahill S, Begley E, Faulkner JP, Hagen I. "It gives me a sense of independence" – findings from Ireland on the use and usefulness of assistive technology for people with dementia. Technol Disabil. 2007;19(2/3):133–42.
21. Scherer MJ, Sax C, Vanbiervliet A, Cushman LA, Scherer JV. Predictors of assistive technology use: the importance of personal and psychosocial factors. Disabil Rehabil. 2005;27(21):1321–31.
22. Scherer MJ, Glueckauf R. Assessing the benefits of assistive technologies for activities and participation. Rehabil Psychol. 2005;50(2):132–41.
23. Scherer MJ. From people-centered to person-centered services, and back again. Disabil Rehabil Assist Technol. 2014;9(1):1–2.
24. Andrich R, Mathiassen NE, Hoogerwerf EJ, Gelderblom GJ. Service delivery systems for assistive technology in Europe: an AAATE/EASTIN position paper. Technol Disabil. 2013;25(3):127–46.
25. Agree EM, Freedman VA. A quality-of-life scale for assistive technology: results of a pilot study of aging and technology. Phys Ther. 2011;91(12):1780–8.
26. Cabrera M, Özcivelek R. ICT for independent living services [Internet]. ResearchGate. [citato 2019 marzo 26]. https://www.researchgate.net/publication/296412185_ICT_for_independent_living_services.
27. National Research Council (US) Steering Committee for the Workshop on Technology for Adaptive Aging, Pew RW, Van Hemel SB. Technology for adaptive aging (The National Academies collection: reports funded by National Institutes of Health). Washington, DC: National Academies Press; 2004 [citato 2019 marzo 26]. http://www.ncbi.nlm.nih.gov/books/NBK97346/.
28. Zabala J, Blunt M, Carl D, Davis S, Deterding C, Foss T, et al. Quality indicators for assistive technology services in school settings. J Spec Educ Technol. 2000;15(4):25–36.
29. Al-Shaqi R, Mourshed M, Rezgui Y. Progress in ambient assisted systems for independent living by the elderly. Springerplus. 2016;5:624.

30. Prescott TJ, Robillard JM. Robotic automation can improve the lives of people who need social care. BMJ. 2019;62:364.
31. Majumder S, Aghayi E, Noferesti M, Memarzadeh-Tehran H, Mondal T, Pang Z, et al. Smart homes for elderly healthcare-recent advances and research challenges. Sensors. 2017;17(11):E2496.
32. Dorsey ER, Topol EJ. State of Telehealth. N Engl J Med. 2016;375(2):154–61.
33. Bujnowska-Fedak MM, Pirogowicz I. Support for e-health services among elderly primary care patients. Telemed J E Health. 2014;20(8):696–704.
34. ICT and ageing - European study on users, markets and technologies. Digital Single Market. [citato 2019 marzo 26]. https://ec.europa.eu/digital-single-market/en/news/ict-and-ageing-european-study-users-markets-and-technologies.
35. Beuscher LM, Fan J, Sarkar N, Dietrich MS, Newhouse PA, Miller KF, et al. Socially assistive robots: measuring older adults' perceptions. J Gerontol Nurs. 2017;43(12):35–43.
36. Vandemeulebroucke T, de Casterlé BD, Gastmans C. How do older adults experience and perceive socially assistive robots in aged care: a systematic review of qualitative evidence. Aging Ment Health. 2018;22(2):149–67.
37. Vaportzis E, Clausen MG, Gow AJ. Older adults perceptions of technology and barriers to interacting with tablet computers: a focus group study. Front Psychol. 2017;8:1687.
38. Rust KL, Smith RO. Assistive technology in the measurement of rehabilitation and health outcomes: a review and analysis of instruments. Am J Phys Med Rehabil. 2005;84(10):780–93; quiz 794–6.
39. Fleming R, Sum S. Empirical studies on the effectiveness of assistive technology in the care of people with dementia: a systematic review [Internet]. York: Centre for Reviews and Dissemination; 2014 [citato 2019 marzo 26]. https://www.ncbi.nlm.nih.gov/books/NBK236935/.
40. Piau A, Campo E, Rumeau P, Vellas B, Nourhashémi F. Aging society and gerontechnology: a solution for an independent living? J Nutr Health Aging. 2014;18(1):97–112.
41. Chung J, Demiris G, Thompson HJ. Ethical considerations regarding the use of smart home technologies for older adults: an integrative review. Annu Rev Nurs Res. 2016;34:155–81.
42. Emiliani PL. Assistive technology (AT) versus mainstream technology (MST): the research perspective. Technol Disabil. 2006;18(1):19–29.
43. Foley A, Ferri BA. Technology for people, not disabilities: ensuring access and inclusion. J Res Spec Educ Needs. 2012;12(4):192–200.
44. Group BMJP. Streptomycin treatment of pulmonary tuberculosis. BMJ. 1998;317(7167):1248.
45. Ligthelm RJ, Borzì V, Gumprecht J, Kawamori R, Wenying Y, Valensi P. Importance of observational studies in clinical practice. Clin Ther. 2007;29:Spec No:1284–92.
46. Sessler DI, Imrey PB. Clinical research methodology 3: randomized controlled trials. Anesth Analg. 2015;121(4):1052–64.
47. Hernandez AF, Fleurence RL, Rothman RL. The ADAPTABLE trial and PCORnet: shining light on a new research paradigm. Ann Intern Med. 2015;163(8):635–6.
48. Lederle FA, Cushman WC, Ferguson RE, Brophy MT, Fiore Md LD. Chlorthalidone versus hydrochlorothiazide: a new kind of veterans affairs cooperative study. Ann Intern Med. 2016;165(9):663–4.
49. Faubion CW, Andrew JD. Book Review: Dillman, D. A. (2000). Mail and internet surveys: the tailored design method (2nd ed.). New York: Wiley 464 pp., $47.50 (hardcover). Rehabil Couns Bull. 2001;44(3):178–80.
50. Higgins JPT, Altman DG, Gøtzsche PC, Jüni P, Moher D, Oxman AD, et al. The Cochrane Collaboration's tool for assessing risk of bias in randomised trials. BMJ. 2011;343:d5928.
51. Holly C, Salmond S, Saimbert M. Comprehensive systematic review for advanced practice nursing. 2nd ed. New York: Springer Publishing Company; 2016. 500 p.
52. Munn Z, Moola S, Riitano D, Lisy K. The development of a critical appraisal tool for use in systematic reviews addressing questions of prevalence. Int J Health Policy Manag. 2014;3(3):123–8.

53. Friedman LM, Furberg CD, DeMets D. Fundamentals of clinical trials [internet]. 4th ed. New York: Springer; 2010. [citato 28 marzo 2019]. https://www.springer.com/la/book/9781441915863.
54. Tomlin G, Borgetto B. Research pyramid: a new evidence-based practice model for occupational therapy. Am J Occup Ther. 2011;65(2):189–96.
55. Kovner AR, Rundall TG. Evidence-based management reconsidered. Front Health Serv Manag. 2006;22(3):3–22.
56. Larzelere RE, Kuhn BR, Johnson B. The intervention selection bias: an underrecognized confound in intervention research. Psychol Bull. 2004;130(2):289–303.
57. Berger VW, Alperson SY. A general framework for the evaluation of clinical trial quality. Rev Recent Clin Trials. 2009;4(2):79–88.
58. Steiner PM, Kim Y, Hall CE, Su D. Graphical models for quasi-experimental designs. Sociol Methods Res. 2017;46(2):155–88.
59. Kim Y, Steiner P. Quasi-Experimental Designs for Causal Inference. Educ Psychol. 2016;51(3–4):395–405.
60. Lee SW, Taylor R, Kielhofner G, Fisher G. Theory use in practice: a national survey of therapists who use the model of human occupation. Am J Occup Ther. 2008;62(1):106–17.
61. Pozzi C, Lanzoni A, Lucchi E, Bergamini L, Bevilacqua P, Manni B, et al. A pilot study of community-based occupational therapy for persons with dementia (COTID-IT program) and their caregivers: evidence for applicability in Italy. Aging Clin Exp Res. 2019;31(9):1299–304. https://doi.org/10.1007/s40520-018-1078-7.
62. Hynes SM, Field B, Ledgerd R, Swinson T, Wenborn J, di Bona L, et al. Exploring the need for a new UK occupational therapy intervention for people with dementia and family carers: community occupational therapy in dementia (COTiD). A focus group study. Aging Ment Health. 2016;20(7):762–9.
63. Wenborn J, Hynes S, Moniz-Cook E, Mountain G, Poland F, King M, et al. Community occupational therapy for people with dementia and family carers (COTiD-UK) versus treatment as usual (valuing active life in dementia [VALID] programme): study protocol for a randomised controlled trial. Trials. 2016;17(1):65.
64. Lanzoni A, Fabbo A, Basso D, Pedrazzini P, Bortolomiol E, Jones M, et al. Interventions aimed to increase independence and Well-being in patients with Alzheimer's disease: review of some interventions in the Italian context. Neurol Psychiatry Brain Res. 2018;30:137–43.

Christian Pozzi is lecturer at the University of Applied Sciences and Arts of Southern Switzerland (SUPSI) and collaborator of the Centre of Competence on Ageing at the same university. He completed his BSc in Occupational Therapy in 2008 and MSc in Physical Education in 2004: for the last 12 years he has worked in the field of rehabilitation. He is President of Argilla Association, a non-profit association. He collaborates with the Geriatric Research Group of Brescia and the Occupational Therapists Association in Italy and Switzerland to promote the inclusion of people with disabilities.

Stefano Cavalli is PhD in sociology, is professor of life course and ageing at the University of Applied Sciences and Arts of Southern Switzerland (SUPSI) and head of the Centre of Competence on Ageing at the same university. He is an expert in sociological research on ageing, with particular focus on transitions and life events in very old age, entry into nursing homes and end-of-life decisions.

Cristian Leorin is an Adjunct Professor at University of Padua and at University of Modena-Reggio Emilia where he teaches and conducts courses on "Assistive Technology and Speech Language Pathology" and "Augmentative and Alternative Communication". In the last 10 years, he also provided consulting services to non-profit and public organizations as an external expert (European Commission, Minister of Health and Regional and Local health Department) involved in developing new services and technologies to improve the quality of life, health and autonomy of individuals (especially elderly, people with disabilities, social disadvantage). He is the President of Novilunio, a non-profit association that in collaboration with medical institutions and industry partners designs and develops experimental projects that promote the adoption of assistive technologies and home modifications in the elderly and people with dementia.

Omar Cauli is Medical Doctor (GP) and Pharmacologist, PhD in Neuroscience, Associate Professor at the Faculty of Nursing and Podology, University of Valencia (Spain). Author of more than 120 scientific publications in journals of recognized international prestige and high-impact factor in the field of Neurology, Geriatrics, Neurosciences, Psychiatry and others. He co-authored a book on the management of extrapyramidal cerebral palsy. His research experience is supported by his participation as an associate and main researcher in 38 research projects funded by Spanish and European Union public entities or private contracts. He co-authored an international patent related to the use of a biomarker to detect cognitive impairment in patients with liver cirrhosis. Reviewer for several scientific projects and articles, and Member of several Editorial Boards and Guest Editor of 4 special issues in high-impact journals.

Alessandro Morandi MD, MPH, is a geriatric consultant at the Department of Rehabilitation and Aged Care Unit of the Ancelle Hospital of the Fondazione Teresa Camplani in Cremona (Italy). He is an adjunct professor at the University of Brescia where he teaches Geriatrics in the Physical Therapists University. He is author of more than 90 scientific publications in international journals. He is an experienced researcher on delirium, geriatric syndromes and geriatric rehabilitation. He is the past president of the European Delirium Association.

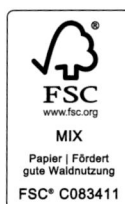

Zeitfracht Medien GmbH
Ferdinand-Jühlke-Straße 7
99095 Erfurt, Deutschland
produktsicherheit@kolibri360.de